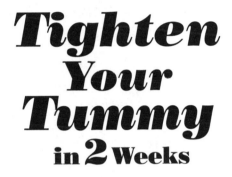

Tighten Your Tummy in 2 Weeks

Other Books by Ellington Darden, PhD

Nutrition and Athletic Performance

How to Lose Body Fat

Especially for Women

Strength-Training Principles

The Athlete's Guide to Sports Medicine

The Nautilus Book

The Nautilus Bodybuilding Book

The Nautilus Diet

The Six-Week Fat-to-Muscle Makeover

Hot Hips and Fabulous Thighs

High-Intensity Bodybuilding

High-Intensity Home Training

Soft Steps to a Hard Body

Living Longer Stronger

Body Defining

A Flat Stomach ASAP

The Bowflex Body Plan

The New Bodybuilding for Old-School Results

The New High Intensity Training

The Body Fat Breakthrough

**LOSE UP TO 14 INCHES
& 14 POUNDS OF FAT
IN 14 DAYS!**

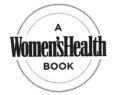

A
Women'sHealth
BOOK

Tighten Your Tummy
in 2 Weeks

ELLINGTON DARDEN, PhD
Author of *The Body Fat Breakthrough*

RODALE.

© 2015 by Ellington Darden, PhD

All rights reserved. No part of this publication may be reproduced or transmitted in any form or by any means, electronic or mechanical, including photocopying, recording, or any other information storage and retrieval system, without the written permission of the publisher.

Rodale books may be purchased for business or promotional use or for special sales. For information, please write to:
Special Markets Department, Rodale Inc., 733 Third Avenue, New York, NY 10017.

Women's Health is a registered trademark of Rodale Inc.

Printed in the United States of America

Rodale Inc. makes every effort to use acid-free ⊗, recycled paper ♺.

Book design by Carol Angstadt

Exercise photographs by Mitch Mandel

Other photos by Ellington Darden, except for page 44, which is by William Boyd.

Illustration on page 25 by Karen Kuchar

Library of Congress Cataloging-in-Publication Data is on file with the publisher.

ISBN-13: 978–1–62336–571–4 hardcover

Distributed to the trade by Macmillan

2   4   6   8   10   9   7   5   3   1   hardcover

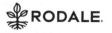

We inspire and enable people to improve their lives and the world around them.
rodalebooks.com

contents

Part I
TIGHTEN YOUR
TUMMY AWARENESS

Part II
THE SCIENCE
OF FAT LOSS

Part III
BEST TUMMY TIGHTENERS

Part IV
THE PROGRAM

Part V
MAINTENANCE AND INSPIRATION

Success Stories

What Women Say after Completing the Tighten Your Tummy Program

"25 inches! My waist hasn't been this small
since I was in the sixth grade."

—*Brianna Kramer,* 23, artist, lost 20 pounds of fat in 6 weeks

"For 27 years, I weighed more than 200 pounds. Thanks
to the Tighten Your Tummy program, I now weigh 152
pounds. It truly has been a life-changing experience."

**—*Katie Smith,* 60, mother of 4, lost
62 pounds of fat in 18 weeks**

"I could never do a single pushup, not ever in my
entire life. Now I can do 10 consecutive ones. Is it
a miracle? No. It's due to Ellington Darden's
negative-accentuated style of exercise."

—*Joan Cortez,* 62, retired teacher, lost 26 pounds in 12 weeks

"I believe Ellington Darden must understand
the science of losing fat and tightening the tummy
better than anyone in the world."

**—*Roxanne Dybevick,* 54, artist, lost 15 pounds
of fat in 2 weeks**

"Now I have a curve in my lower back, right above my
jeans, that makes me look so much more shapely. Plus,
I have found my cheek and collarbones."

**—*Jennifer MacCallum,* 34, mother of 4,
lost 34 pounds in 12 weeks**

"With the stress of everyday life, I so often do not feel in control. Completing the Tighten Your Tummy program has made me feel very much in control of my life . . . and happy."

—*Julie Hill,* **64, executive director, lost 18 pounds of fat in 6 weeks**

"I am fitting into jeans I never thought I would again. My husband tells me how slender I look. I am very pleased."

—*Joyce Dorval,* **61, real estate broker, lost 20 pounds of fat in 6 weeks**

"I feel amazing. I love the person I now see in the mirror."

—*Laura Morrow,* **30, attorney, mother of 2, lost 21 pounds of fat in 6 weeks**

"As a vegetarian, I had no trouble adapting the Tighten Your Tummy plan. My waistline got smaller with each passing week and my stomach muscles got stronger."

—*Sara Smith,* **64, monkey caregiver at primate sanctuary, lost 14 total inches from her waist in 2 weeks**

Comments are from participants in Ellington Darden's Tighten Your Tummy test program at Gainesville Health & Fitness in 2014.

Now, How About YOU?

BEFORE & AFTER 16 WEEKS

Jeanenne Darden
Age 54 • Height 5 feet, 7.5 inches

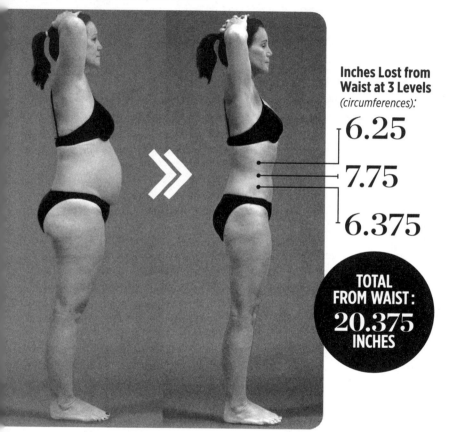

Inches Lost from Waist at 3 Levels
(circumferences):

6.25

7.75

6.375

TOTAL FROM WAIST:
20.375
INCHES

Weight Before: **184.5 pounds**
Weight After: **148 pounds**
FAT LOSS: 40.5 pounds
Muscle Gain: **4 pounds**

"Commit to 2 weeks,
SERIOUSLY,
and it will change
your life!"
—*Jeanenne Darden*

introduction

A Life Saved... A Body Transformed

How You Too Can Lose and Rebuild

"My middle is a mess. From the side, my body looks like a barrel."

That's what my wife said to me one morning in the fall of 2013 as she saw her reflection in our full-length mirror. "Please help me ... NOW," Jeanenne pleaded.

I had been trying to convince her to do my basic diet and exercise program, which she knew by heart, especially since she'd started and stopped it three or four times in the last year. But on that day, I knew she was at the end of her rope, that she was absolutely serious.

Over the last two years, Jeanenne had gone through a series of life-threatening experiences. In March 2011, while vacationing in Aruba, she nearly drowned. She was swimming in the ocean with our 6-year-old daughter riding on her back. Jeanenne is a strong swimmer, but she suddenly started gasping for air and going under. Luckily, our friend Gregg Godlewski, a former lifeguard, spotted her struggling and was able to rescue her.

Something, however, wasn't right in her chest. She flew back home to Orlando the next morning, where doctors told her she was in congestive heart failure; blood was regurgitating back into her upper heart chamber. She needed to be operated on immediately.

Two days later, Jeanenne had open-heart surgery to repair a mitral valve that wouldn't close. For the second time in a week, her life had been saved.

Saved but Not Better

The recovery was slow and fraught with complications, like a grapefruit-size blood clot that required more surgery and caused extreme pain for 2 weeks. She stopped all exercise. She then started a medication that caused her to gain weight. Over the next 6 months, she put on 40 pounds, making her the heaviest she'd ever been, at 184.5 pounds.

My wife has always been lean and athletic. She had natural childbirths at ages 42 and 45. Even during pregnancy, her friends would say, "Gosh, Jeanenne, your arms and shoulders look amazing." Exercise and active living are an integral part of her life. We have a full gym in our home, but Jeanenne could no longer bring herself to use it. "I was so depressed thinking I'd never be the same," she remembered. "I love clothes and dressing, but none of them fit anymore. I started to hate myself."

I knew right then, in front of our full-length mirror, that my wife needed help and that I had to have a no-fail solution.

A New Program

I was very relieved when Jeanenne asked for my help, because it demonstrated her first steps toward coming out of the depression that had paralyzed her after surgery. I was worried about her, but this was a good sign; she realized she needed to work toward gaining back some control in her life. And for me it meant that I was on the path to gaining back the woman I knew and loved.

For months before Jeanenne's health problems began, I had been researching a new approach to eliminating belly fat. It occurred to me that Jeanenne would be the ideal subject to test my theories. Like many women who go through a physical or emotional challenge in middle age, she gained a significant amount of weight and lost both muscle and her fitness level. She was depressed and unhappy with herself. She needed a plan that would show quick, positive results to lift her spirits and motivate her to keep moving forward.

I knew I was on to something when Jeanenne lost 10 pounds during the first 2 weeks on my diet and exercise program. Ten pounds in just 14 days! Those quick results gave Jeanenne the confidence and resolve to stay the course through some of the most difficult times of her life and the most challenging times of the year to embark on a diet, namely Halloween, Thanksgiving, Christmas, New Year's, and Valentine's Day!

Jeanenne prevailed triumphantly. She emerged from her "barrel" in March 2014 more than 40 pounds lighter, with a brand-new body and her confidence back. Her life—thanks to her doggedly determined work ethic—had been not only saved, but also quite literally transformed for the better.

Several components of the program led to Jeanenne's success, but one was especially powerful and really surprised her—and may surprise you, too. What is it? Extra sleep. That's right, getting extra sleep proved to be a critical component to Jeanenne's success, and that's why it's an important part of the Tighten Your Tummy in 2 Weeks program. You'll read the details in Chapter 11.

Throughout November, December, and January, whenever Jeanenne felt the urge to eat high-calorie foods, she took a nap. Or at night, when her appetite surged, she retired to bed early. That way, she avoided consuming extra dietary calories and, with close attention given to the Tighten Your Tummy diet, she burned calories as she slept.

You Can Snooze to Lose?

Snooze to Lose. That's what Jeanenne and I named this concept. Most people don't realize that during a diet program more than 50 percent of the fat loss occurs while you sleep.

Equally important is that 99 percent of the strength- and muscle-building process from an intense exercise session takes place—again—*while you are sleeping.* So more sleep also equals more effective muscle building.

(continued on page xvi)

GET YOUR BEST BODY BACK

Start seeing results with a 2-week committment

MY FAVORITE SKINNY JEANS DIDN'T FIT. Forget the top button. I couldn't get the leg holes to go over my thighs. I felt like crying . . . again.

I know how it feels to go into a closet and stare at all the clothes that used to fit. Have you been there, too? I had nothing to wear—because I couldn't squeeze into anything. I felt terrible. I had admitted defeat and finally went shopping for a few things that I could put on, just so I'd have something to wear. I remember the feeling of seeing a large, overfat version of myself—and then thinking, "I'll never get my lean body back." I know the feeling of wanting the fat off *now*!

That's exactly what I experienced on October 14, 2013. I decided right then to commit completely to my husband Ell's new program.

Two weeks later, I was down 10 pounds. I was thrilled. I could feel the results and see the difference. It was just the success I needed to commit to another 2 weeks. The more I lost, the more disciplined I was in following the program. I was determined to not let any holiday or special occasion sabotage my progress.

A stronger, leaner me began to emerge, and I began to like what I was seeing in the mirror. I was getting my body, and my life, back. And my favorite jeans now fit the way they're supposed to. Thank goodness!

You can get your best body back too with Ellington's Tighten Your Tummy program. My before-and-after photos prove how effective it is, but if you still can't believe the author's wife, well, consider the testimonials of the 41 other women who have experienced dramatic success in this book. Then try it yourself: Commit to just 2 weeks. The results you achieve will give you the momentum to go another 2 weeks and then another and however longer you need to reach your goal.

Before you know it, you'll be back in your closet with plenty of options—including that sexy pair of skinny jeans. Good luck. I know you'll do great!

—*Jeanenne*

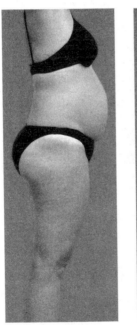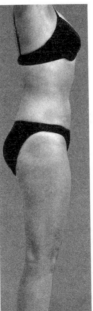

These before-and-after photos of Jeanenne Darden show exactly where she lost the inches, which totaled 42.875 from eight locations on the tummy, hips, and thighs.

Extra sleep, reduced-calorie eating, and strength training were three of the five essential components in Jeanenne's success. The fourth was a mini exercise called the inner-ab vacuum, which she practiced before each meal. The fifth was superhydration: drinking a gallon of ice water every day. Together, these five components formed a dynamic, unbeatable weight-loss strategy.

Burn Belly Fat

If you are a woman between 18 and 80 years of age who wants to lose 10 to 20 pounds of fat, especially the flab around your tummy, then look no further. You're holding in your hands a unique plan to burn belly fat and strengthen the midsection muscles quickly, in 2 to 6 weeks. The most fat that any of my test panel women lost in 2 weeks was 15 pounds, so if you have more than 15 pounds to remove—perhaps as much as 20 to 30 pounds—it's going to require at least 6 weeks or longer. Applied properly, this program could transform your body like never before, just as it did for my wife and for the other women you will meet in this book.

This extraordinary course, and its no-fail solution, will absolutely work for you. With your commitment to following these science-backed strategies, you will start seeing significant improvements in your body in just days and certainly within the first 2 weeks.

Please note: The eating plan in *Tighten Your Tummy in 2 Weeks* is designed for women. The dietary calories each day are too low for most men.

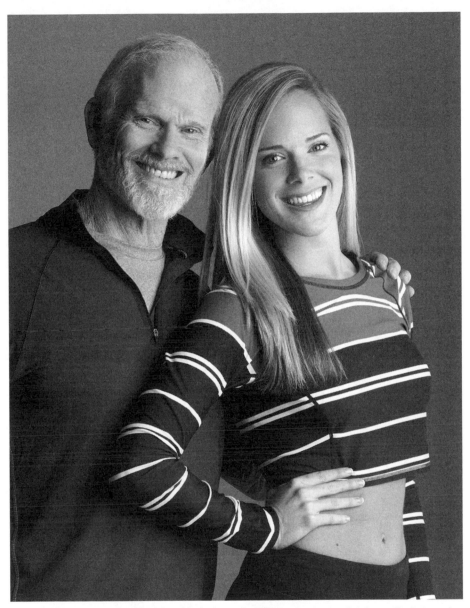

My daughter Sarah made such great progress on the Tighten Your Tummy program that she's featured in photographs throughout the book and demonstrates the exercises in Chapter 10. Thank you, Sarah, for all your dedicated effort.

Part I
TIGHTEN YOUR TUMMY AWARENESS

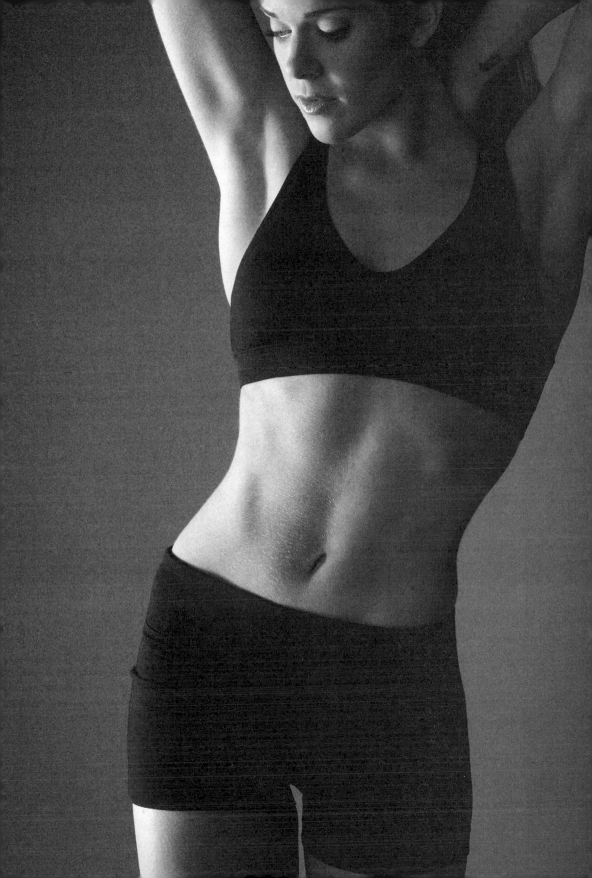

BEFORE & AFTER 12 WEEKS

Sarah Darden
Age 25 • Height 5 feet, 7.5 inches

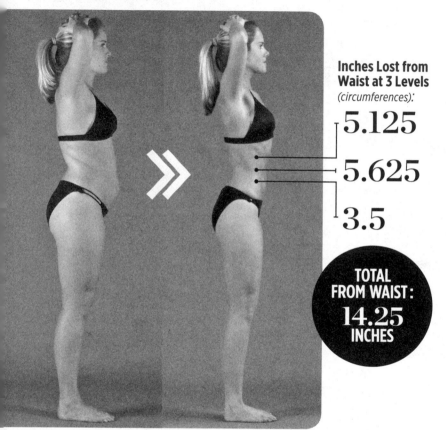

Inches Lost from Waist at 3 Levels
(circumferences):

5.125

5.625

3.5

TOTAL FROM WAIST:
14.25
INCHES

Weight Before: **158.6 pounds**

Weight After: **135.1 pounds**

FAT LOSS: 26.86 pounds

Muscle Gain: **3.36 pounds**

"My job put the pounds on. I needed some structure in my life to slim down."

—Sarah Darden

chapter

1

Where Does Beauty Begin?

History Has Some Surprising Answers

In 2015, for the first time, *Sports Illustrated*'s annual swimsuit issue showcased a plus-size model, Ashley Graham. It was bold. It was refreshing to see. And it was an anomaly. From Victoria's Secret Fashion Shows to *ESPN*'s "Body" editions to TV commercials for automobiles, lean midsections and flat stomachs are used to help market products. You'll see a few male models with six-pack abs hawking underwear, but for the most part, advertising focuses its selling attention on the female midriff.

Of course, beauty contests, which feature women in bathing suits and bikinis, have been a staple in the United States for more than 75 years. And men's magazines, such as *Playboy*—which displays scantily clad Playmates each month—have been in circulation for almost as long. The vast majority of the contest winners and the monthly cover girls are taller than average and have smaller-than-average waistlines, according to Will Lassek, MD, assistant professor of epidemiology at the University of Pittsburgh. In his article titled "Eternal Curves," published online at *Psychology Today,* he noted that American men spend $3 billion a year to gaze at women with curvy hips that taper into small, flat waists.

Why all the fascination with female flat bellies?

Clues, Concepts, and Answers

A scientist named Devendra Singh, PhD, who grew up in Urai, India, spent his entire academic career searching for answers to that question. A professor of psychology at the University of Texas for four decades, he pioneered the field of evolutionary psychology. The late Dr. Singh's most notable research dealt with the historical significance of a woman's waist-to-hip ratio from the standpoint of health, attractiveness, and reproduction.

In his experiments, Dr. Singh asked groups of men and women to rank a series of 12 figure drawings showing various sizes and curves of waists and hips. He found that both groups were most attracted to the "hourglass shape" of the body and determined from the survey the optimal waist-to-hip ratio. In other analysis, he discovered that seeing a female with that optimal waist-to-hip ratio activates pleasure centers in the brains of men, the same areas of the prefrontal cortex and hypothalamus targeted by cocaine and heroin. Dr. Singh found that in social interactions, for example, a man quickly eyes a woman from top to bottom and then zeros in on the midsection. He makes a primal evaluation—*attractive* or *not attractive, interested* or *not interested*—in a split second, without even being aware of the judgment he's making.

But why is a male attracted to an hourglass figure in the first place? Dr. Singh methodically traced the answer back some 200,000 years. Our cave-dwelling ancestors had to be seriously tough, as well as alert and fast acting. There were no high-tech diagnostic tools or miracle drugs to correct broken bones or fight infections. Sickness or injury meant disability and being left behind. Wild animals were always a threat. Drought and volatile weather brought starvation and death. These constant threats of danger made survival a man's primary preoccupation.

Gradually, the prehistoric man learned that his only viable means of gene survival was to sire healthy children *repeatedly*. To produce healthy children, he had to find and mate with healthy, fertile women. In a caveman's mind, a big-bellied woman was either pregnant, which meant unavailable for mating, or overweight and fat, which meant unhealthy (or not fit enough to outrun a saber-toothed tiger). The only way to be sure his sperm had its best shot at producing offspring was to search for that hourglass shape with a flat tummy that signified "I'm fit and fertile."

Fertility and Genetic Longevity

After taking thousands of waist and hip measurements and scaling their ratios, Dr. Singh determined that the perfect female waist measures 25.25 inches and hips measure 36 inches. Those numbers, 25.25/36, equal a waist-to-hip ratio of 0.7; stated another way, the hip measurement is 1.4 times larger than the waist. Want a contemporary example of a nearly perfect waist-to-hip ratio? Check out Jennifer Lopez in her 2014 "Booty" video. With a flat middle and ample booty, J.Lo has the best of both body parts.

Interestingly, paintings from the Renaissance period from the 14th through the 17th centuries depict women with plump bodies, much heavier than the 20th-century ideal. But according to Dr. Singh, the waist-to-hip ratio shown in those works of art was still 0.7. Even the paintings of the plump Greek goddess Aphrodite, from more than 1,000 years earlier, had a similar 0.7 waist-to-hip ratio. To the artist's eye, this ratio was perfection.

During the 1920s, the popular flapper-style dresses tended to cover the body in a more tubular fashion, suggesting an androgynous body shape. Still, the most attractive models and celebrities of that day had hourglass figures. The same thing occurred during the 1970s, when British models exhibited a tubular style of dress. Hidden underneath those straight lines were women with small waists and curvy hips. In fact, when men and women were asked to rank beauty from a lineup of body shapes, tubular-shaped women were considered unattractive. This was true not only in the United States but in almost all countries surveyed.

Another key evolutionary part of the attraction game is symmetry. Both men and women (and most other animals) are more attracted to faces and bodies that are more symmetrical. So it stands to reason that any excessive characteristic (like a fat tummy) that makes the human form less than symmetrical would be considered less attractive. The vital lesson from history is: A woman's waist-to-hip ratio makes a significant difference. Beauty does begin with a flat stomach.

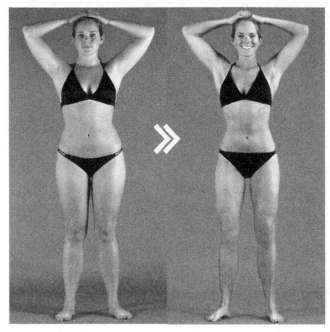

My daughter Sarah Darden was delighted with her Tighten Your Tummy results. Besides losing 14.25 inches off her waist, she dropped 4 inches off her hips and 6.125 inches off her thighs. Plus, her waist-to-hip ratio was smaller (which means more hourglass) than 0.7 at 24.5/36.75 = 0.67.

Lana, Ava, and Liz Had It . . .

So did Marilyn, Sophia, and Brigitte!

Dr. Singh summarized that no matter the era, the icons of beauty have consistently had waist-to-hip ratios of approximately 0.7. Whether they were classified as underweight, normal weight, or overweight, the recognized stars of yesterday and today fit the mold: Lana Turner, Ava Gardner, Esther Williams, Elizabeth Taylor, Grace Kelly, Marilyn Monroe, Sophia Loren, Brigitte Bardot, Twiggy, Jane Fonda, Keira Knightley, Jennifer Aniston, and Taylor Swift each had or have that magic ratio.

You can, too. Even if you believe you are "big boned" or if you are a large woman and have significant fat on your body, you can achieve that attractive hourglass shape by tightening your tummy. And the benefits go far beyond appearance. A flat stomach helps protect women from an array of diseases ranging from diabetes, hypertension, heart attack, stroke, osteoarthritis, and even depression.

Happiness Is Contagious

We may not wish to admit it, but being happy with the shape and look of our bodies can have a significant positive effect on our outlook on life. If you are unhappy with the shape of your midsection, as many people are, I believe that tightening your tummy can help you feel happier and more confident. Certainly achieving a fitness goal like a flatter belly can prove to you that you can do anything you set your mind to. It happened to the 41 overweight women in my test panels at Gainesville Health & Fitness. When a woman loses 8 to 15 pounds of fat in 2 weeks—and as much as 10 to 14 inches off her waist at three levels—her self-esteem goes sky-high and her happiness abounds.

"I love the person I have become," 30-year-old participant Laura Morrow told me.

"I feel really good about myself," said Nannette Carnes, the oldest woman in the Tighten Your Tummy program at 79!

Their happiness can be contagious. So honor the hourglass figure hidden within you. Welcome to the Tighten Your Tummy in 2 Weeks program. I look forward to hearing about your success.

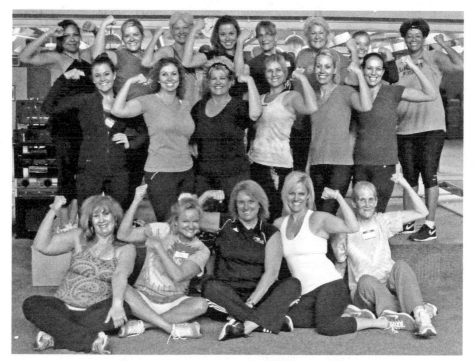

The Tighten Your Tummy test panel was split into two groups of 20 and 21 women, respectively. In Group 1, the average age, height, and starting body weight was 47.4 years, 66.8 inches, and 163.7 pounds. As a group, they lost 289 pounds of fat in 6 weeks and more than 214 inches off their waists. They also built 60 pounds of lean muscle and earned the right to show it off.

BEFORE & AFTER 6 WEEKS

Laura Morrow
Age 30 • Height 5 feet, 5.5 inches

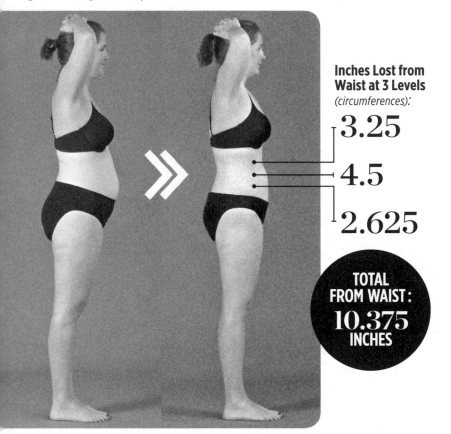

Inches Lost from Waist at 3 Levels
(*circumferences*):

3.25

4.5

2.625

TOTAL FROM WAIST:

10.375 INCHES

Weight Before: **161.9 pounds**

Weight After: **144.8 pounds**

FAT LOSS: 21.59 pounds

Muscle Gain: **4.49 pounds**

"The program kept my enthusiasm moving higher, as my waistline was shrinking lower."

—*Laura Morrow*

chapter
2
How to Tighten Your Tummy

The Five-Part Formula for Success

Okay, you want a flat stomach. Here's a question for you: Can you remember the last time you actually had one? What was the year?

Were you in the seventh grade? Was it after dance camp or when you graduated from high school or just before you married? Was it before your first pregnancy? Close your eyes and visualize this time and what it meant to you. You looked good and felt good, didn't you? In those days, without being conscious of it, you probably had a lean and tight middle. You could eat just about anything you wanted and not get fat, or so it seemed. Now, however, things have changed.

Look down at your navel. Has it gradually disappeared from view? Do rolls of flab surround it? Is there a pouch of fat under it? When you hear those "muffin top" references, are you afraid you qualify? Has it been some time since you buttoned the top of your jeans? Don't beat yourself up. There's a reason many of us put on weight as the years pass. As we age, our metabolism slows, and we lose some muscle mass (a big burner of calories). On top of that, high-calorie foods are everywhere. The abundance of cheap food adds to our challenge to stay lean. A lot of women—check that, *most* women—are in the same boat as you.

Maybe you'd just like to lose a few pounds and inches off your waistline so your clothes will look and feel better. Maybe you want to reduce your belly and elsewhere because you have a wedding or reunion coming up in a few months. Maybe you are concerned about your health and know that eliminating dangerous fat from around your internal organs is one of the best ways to reduce your risk of diabetes, heart disease, and cancer. Whether you want to lose a little or a lot, if you identified with any of the above statements, Tighten Your Tummy in 2 Weeks is the program for you.

DEFINING YOUR MIDDLE

TUMMY, WAIST, BELLY, STOMACH, MIDSECTION, ABS, and *core* have all been used to mean the area of the human body below the ribs and above the hips. Generally, the *waist* refers to the smallest circumference measurement in inches between the ribs and hips. *Tummy* and *stomach* can mean the initial organ of digestion, as well as the front of the waist.

Midsection is the middle region of the human torso. *Abs* refers to the rectus abdominis, which are long, flat muscles on the front torso and are separated by a midline band of connective tissue. Fully developed, the rectus abdominis muscles are often called the six-pack. *Core* is a recent term that means midsection and usually includes the deeper muscles supporting the spine and pelvic girdle.

Chapter 1 introduced you to some evolutionary reasons for a flat stomach. Now I'm going to share with you some statistics, several scientific discussion points, and notes about my test panel of 41 women that will help you understand why the Tighten Your Tummy program is so effective.

How Women Feel about Their Tummies

Glamour magazine's November 2014 issue reported a revealing survey titled "How Do You Feel about Your Body?" *Glamour* surveyed 1,000 women between 18 and 40 years of age. The 2014 results were then compared to a similar study of women conducted by the same magazine in 1984.

The 1984 survey showed that 41 percent of the women polled were unhappy with their bodies. The most-hated body part? The thighs, with 72 percent saying that they felt "ashamed" of theirs. Some 30 years later, you might expect women to show improvement in their self-acceptance. After all, women have made such great strides, rising to the top in every field imaginable. Unfortunately, as confident and successful as women have become from the battlefields to the boardrooms, that's not the case when it comes to body confidence.

In 2014, 54 percent of women polled—13 percent more than in 1984—reported being unhappy with their body. Another statistic changed: The most hated body part in 2014 became the tummy or belly, with 76 percent admitting to being unhappy with and ashamed of their midsection. According to the author, Shaun Dreisbach, tummies have replaced thighs because of an unprecedented parade of skimpy bikini photos online.

The women in *Glamour*'s survey said they spent an average of 2 hours a day on social media alone. The sheer amount of online exposure is staggering: Every day, 1.8 billion photos are uploaded and shared on Facebook, Flickr, Instagram, Snapchat, and WhatsApp. The overriding concern seems to be that women across the board use social media for validation from other women "liking" or "pinning" their photos. Such a need for validation occurs not so much from looking at celebrity pictures, but from poring over photos of friends in revealing outfits and frequently comparing body parts.

Good News

Experts interviewed for the *Glamour* article and many other reported stories about body image suggest that comparing one's body to others', especially on social media, is psychologically unhealthy and unproductive unless you can find a way to use it as motivation to improve. I commend *Glamour*'s editors for encouraging strength over contoured body parts. But the truth is, you can have both. How? First, stop comparing yourself to others. Instead, every day give your body and mind some TLC. Respect your body and its remarkable ability to become stronger and leaner. Try to strengthen your body by exercising properly every week. Be kind to yourself. That means being patient. Every day, tell yourself that you have the power to do anything you put your mind to. With that positive attitude and consistent effort, you can become a leaner, healthier, happier version of yourself.

Tighten Your Tummy in 2 Weeks will be your constant companion to help you reach your goal. My program will strengthen your major muscles and sharpen and contour your waist, hips, thighs, torso, and arms. You will conquer the two major concerns that most women have about their body: weighing less and having a smaller waist.

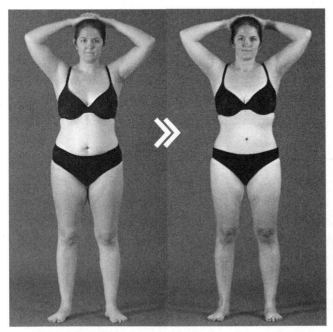

Laura Morrow, an attorney in Gainesville, enthusiastically adopted the strategies in the Power-Start Diet in Chapter 14 and lost 11.5 pounds of fat and 8.375 inches from her waist . . . in just 2 weeks.

Heavy Statistics

A 1996 Harris Poll revealed that 74 percent of American women age 25 and older were overweight. There had been a steady climb from 58 percent in 1983 to 64 percent in 1990 and 71 percent in 1995. Researchers at the time suggested that if this rate of expansion continued unabated, all adult women in the United States would be overweight by the year 2021.

Here's a little bit of good news: Harris Polls taken yearly between 2006 and 2014 show that the percentage of overweight women has finally plateaued, but at 80 percent of the adult population! That's right, four out of every five women living in the United States are overweight—and it has been that way for the past 8 years.

A protruding belly is a key indicator of too much overall body fat. Since there is a high correlation between obesity and belly fat, it stands to reason that you must lose fat throughout your body in order to tighten your tummy. That's exactly what this program will help you to do.

Body Weight and Body Fat

Yes, there's a distinction. When you talk about how much you weigh or how much weight you lost, you're talking about *body weight.* This is the total weight of your unclothed body and is made up of (1) bones, (2) organs (including skin), (3) muscles, and (4) fat. You don't want to be losing weight from all four of these areas. That's a bad thing. What you should be trying to do is lose just the fourth one, *body fat.*

But how do you do that? How do you lose fat and not subtract from the other three components? I've helped people to do that successfully for the last four decades. I do it by teaching how to measure your body fat and how to prevent the loss of fluids from your muscles, organs, and bones. That's all explained in this book. In Chapter 13, I'll show you how to quickly measure your skin-fold thickness and plug that measurement into a formula to find your percentage of body fat.

To prevent the loss of fluids from your muscles, organs, and bones, you must pay close attention to your dietary calories and meal composition—and you must strength-train your body by accentuating the negative part, or lowering, of the movement on a few basic exercises. You'll learn how to eat for a flatter tummy in Chapter 6. The strength-training program is outlined in Chapter 10. Not only do you need to preserve the amount of muscle you have, you need to increase it—and significantly, by 3, 4, 5, and even more pounds of solid muscle.

Finally, a big component of the Tighten Your Tummy plan is getting ample amounts of rest and sleep. By following these guidelines, you will ensure that all your weight loss comes from your fat, not your muscle. Doing so will put you on the road to leanness, strength, and a much tighter tummy.

Muscle-Fat Cross Talk: The Possibility of Spot Reduction

In 2012, I tested a new program I'd created, called the Body Fat Breakthrough, on 145 subjects at the Gainesville Health & Fitness center in Florida. I began to notice that most of the test panel subjects were losing a disproportionate number of inches from their waistlines. It took a while to figure out why. The *why* is related to *muscle-fat cross talk*.

Muscle-fat cross talk is scientific terminology for the interacting chemistry that occurs inside your working muscles as a result of a type of exercise called *negative-accentuated training*. My special type of negative-accentuated exercises for your midsection, combined with the other factors in this program, activate hormones that promote building muscle and mobilizing fat simultaneously.

I began to think, "Maybe it's possible, within certain limitations, to spot-reduce certain areas of your midsection." A more complete discussion of the how-tos of negative-accentuated exercise is found in Chapter 10.

The Inch-by-Inch Loss of Belly Fat

Most weight-loss researchers use a plastic tape to measure a subject's waist in just one location, usually at the navel level or at the smallest position, which is slightly above the navel. A typical "before" waist measurement for a woman might be 30.5 inches. Six weeks later, after losing 10 pounds, that same measurement might be 29 inches. So the woman has reduced the size of her waist by 1.5 inches.

I do things differently. In the last two decades of putting test panelists through weight-loss programs, I've taken the waist measurement at three levels: 2 inches above the navel, at the navel, and 2 inches below the navel (see photos below). You should do the same when you start the program.

Why three levels? Because I've found that some people lose fat faster above the navel, some remove it quicker below the navel, and others notice a difference initially right at navel level. That's especially true for women. By taking measurements from three different locations, you get a more accurate picture of how the diet and exercise program is affecting your body.

Record these three measurements at the beginning of your program, after 2 weeks, and then at the end of 6 weeks. You may notice remarkable results after just 2 weeks, as I did with some of the Tighten Your Tummy participants:

- Marlene Hill, 59, at a starting body weight of 157.7 pounds, stored most of her belly fat well above the navel. She lost 13.23 pounds of fat, and her three waist measurements decreased by 3.5, 3.25, and 3.25 inches.

- Joan Cortez, a 62-year-old mother of two, at a starting body weight of 197 pounds, lost 11.43 pounds of fat and even higher numbers from her waist: 4.75, 5, and 3.75. That's 13.5 inches dropped in only 2 weeks.

- And then there was Sara Smith. At 64, Sara was one of the most dedicated to the program. In just 14 days, she lost 14.125 inches from her waist, with losses at the three sites as follows:

    - *2 inches above the navel: 3.5 inches*
    - *At the navel: 5.125 inches*
    - *2 inches below the navel: 5.5 inches*

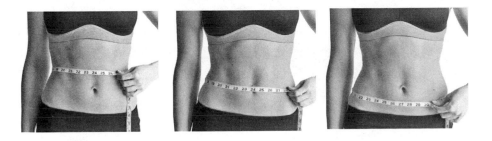

Sara and Joan were number one and two in inches lost from the waist in 2 weeks. Though not in the top 5, Marlene lost more fat. Their rankings reinforce the importance of taking and comparing measurements at the three levels.

The Tighten Your Tummy Test Panel

All 41 women in my Tighten Your Tummy test panels were members of Gainesville Health & Fitness. This is the largest fitness center in the United States, with more than 30,000 members. You can expect to see 5,000 to 6,000 people working out each day.

I've had a great relationship with Joe Cirulli, who has owned and managed the fitness center for more than 30 years. Over the last three decades, I've conducted more than two dozen research projects at the center, all of which involved test panels of subjects. In the fall of 2014, I organized two groups of overfat women who volunteered to be subjects. Each group contained a wide variety of sizes and shapes. Pam Harrison, a personal trainer at the center, and I supervised these two groups through carefully crafted 6-week programs.

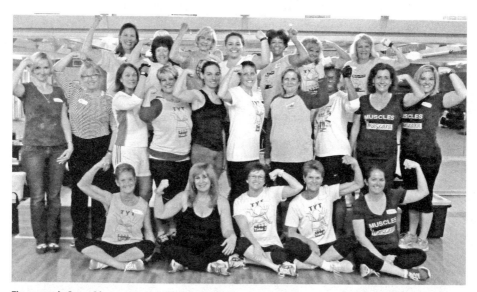

The women in Group 2 lost an average of 16.88 pounds of fat and gained an average of 3.17 pounds of muscle.

ESCAPE THE "ABDOMINAL OBESITY ZONE"

ACCORDING TO THE CENTERS FOR DISEASE Control and Prevention, the size of the average woman's waist grew from 36.3 inches to 37.8 inches from 1999 to 2012. The result is that 64 percent of American women have now moved into what's known as the "abdominal obesity zone." Bellies that big are linked with increased risk of diabetes, heart disease, and premature death.

Many doctors and researchers believe that apathy is one of the chief reasons that many middle-aged women are not taking steps to reduce their belly size. Until they care, really care, experts say, not much is going to change for the better.

But there's good news that should encourage you to take action. The Tighten Your Tummy program really works to maximize fat loss over the entire body, which in turn reduces inches off the waist. With appropriate action, from 37.8 inches, the average woman's waist could quickly shrink down to 34.8 inches. That's 3 inches gone from the navel area circumference, plus another 2.5 inches above the navel and another 2.5 inches below the navel, for a grand total of 8 inches—in only 14 days. This is not unrealistic at all. In fact, it's highly likely, since almost 50 percent of the 41 women in my test panel did just that.

If you are not already serious about getting rid of any excess fat you have around your midsection, then now is the time to take action. In a matter of weeks at least, or months at most, you can escape the "abdominal obesity zone." Soon you'll have leaner, stronger abdominals.

Why don't you make a commitment right now?

You're going to meet many of these women in this book, including Katie Smith, 60, who is the mother of four children. In January 2013, Katie and her husband were involved in an automobile collision that left her with a broken sternum, four broken ribs, and a fractured hip and foot. After months of physical therapy, her progress was poor, and she walked with a limp and had to take all sorts of pain medications just to move around.

Then she joined the Tighten Your Tummy program. After 6 weeks, Katie now walks without a limp, navigates stairs without holding on to the rail, and can pick up and hold her grandkids with ease. She's also 21 pounds lighter—and is embarking on another 6-week session. "This program," Katie says, "changed my life and has given me a future."

Katie's 34-year-old daughter, Jennifer MacCallum, participated too and lost 19 pounds of fat in 6 weeks. "For the first time since I was in high school, I feel confident in wearing a tank top, as well as participating in outdoor activities with my kids," says Jennifer.

Then there's Roxanne Dybevick, 54, who started the program with a 36-inch waist. Roxanne is an artist who sells oil paintings at weekend festivals throughout the South. She subtracted 11.25 inches from her waist during the first 2 weeks and firmed and reshaped her body. Roxanne kept a detailed journal during her Tighten Your Tummy experience. I've included it in Chapter 18; it is enlightening and inspiring.

My 25-year-old daughter, Sarah, was also a test panel subject. Sarah had been active in high school and college and participated on swim teams for many years. She was always lean and in great shape. But then she took her first permanent job as a marketing executive for the Bayfront Auditorium in Pensacola, Florida. During her first year, she put on a good 20 pounds of fat. I knew Sarah had the drive to do my Tighten Your Tummy course on her own in Pensacola. True to form, she was one of the top finishers in her group. You can see her results in photos throughout the book, including demonstrating the exercises in Chapter 10.

A Five-Part Formula for Success

In this chapter, I've discussed the problems associated with a fat, protruding belly and the opportunity for you to become leaner, fitter, and healthier by tightening your tummy. And you've met a few of my test panelists. Their success can be your success if you follow my Tighten Your Tummy program, which is based on this scientific, five-part formula:

1. Two 30-minute strength-training workouts per week using a unique negative-accentuated method of exercising. It involves three 15-second half repetitions, immediately followed by 8 to 12 faster movements. Slower negative-accentuated exercise combined with faster negative-accentuated repetitions is the best way to strengthen and define your abdominal region, as well as other muscles.

   This combination negative exercise style also makes a deeper inroad into your body's starting strength, which in turn triggers at least six hormones that cause your involved midsection muscles to pull calories from surrounding adipose tissue to help fat loss and muscle gain.

2. The "inner-ab vacuum," a technique that, when practiced twice before each meal, strengthens the transverse abdominis muscle. Strengthening this muscle gives a woman more control over her stomach fullness, appetite, and posture.

3. A simple, carbohydrate-rich eating plan that initially reduces then gradually adds calories from basic foods. A key guideline is to eat five or six small meals per day.

4. Extra rest. It is critical to get $8\frac{1}{2}$ hours of sleep each night, plus a 30-minute nap each afternoon. Extra sleep and rest are important because more than 50 percent of fat loss occurs during sleep, and 99 percent of muscle building takes place at night.

5. Superhydration. Sipping ice-cold water continuously throughout the day (a total of a gallon of water per day) synergizes your exercising, eating, and sleeping to accelerate tummy tightening.

BEFORE & AFTER 6 WEEKS

Lynn James
Age 61 • Height 5 feet, 8 inches

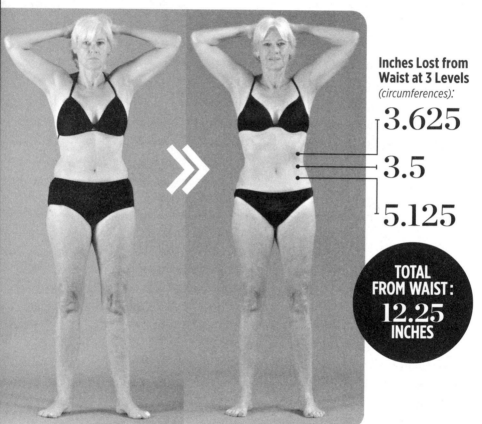

Inches Lost from Waist at 3 Levels
(circumferences):

3.625

3.5

5.125

TOTAL FROM WAIST: 12.25 INCHES

Weight Before: **143 pounds**
Weight After: **131.6 pounds**
FAT LOSS: 14.65 pounds
Muscle Gain: **3.25 pounds**

"I'm now much more conscious of my muscle-to-fat ratio, and I want more muscle!"

—*Lynn James*

chapter
3
Melt Fat All Day and Night

How? Make Some Muscle

Muscle is a critical part of losing weight and staying lean. To get rid of the soft, flabby feel around your midsection and to create tighter, firmer, harder-looking thighs, arms, shoulders, and hips, you need more muscle. That's right, more muscle is your ticket to the body you want.

Some of the women involved in the Tighten Your Tummy program were initially afraid of doing strength-training exercises because they worried about bulking up like a bodybuilder. It's a common fear. A lot of women believe that lifting weights will give them Incredible Hulk muscles. Rest assured, that's not going to happen to you on this program. Instead, you will build lean, well-toned, beautiful muscles that you'll want to show off in a strapless dress. At the end of 6 weeks in my program, all of the women who initially feared the dumbbell had embraced it and built 3 to 4 pounds of muscle. And then they wanted more!

Muscle, the bulging kind that made Arnold Schwarzenegger an action movie star, has been terribly misunderstood. You never have to worry about turning into the Terminator from strength training because you are a woman, and most women are genetically incapable of growing huge, bulging muscles (more on that later). But you can certainly take advantage of the other benefits of strength training. Below are three important reasons that you need more muscle.

1. Muscle Burns Calories

Add 1 pound of muscle to your body and you raise your resting metabolic rate per day by 37.5 calories. Resting metabolic rate is the number of calories that your body burns daily in a relaxed state. An average woman, for example, might have a resting metabolic rate of 1,200 calories per day. Add a pound of muscle and her rate would be raised to 1,237.5 calories per day. Again, that's resting metabolic rate, the amount you would burn, say, while lounging on the couch or sleeping.

Each woman in my Tighten Your Tummy program averaged 3.15 pounds of additional muscle. That amounted to a daily increase of 118.125 calories, which is a significant elevation of energy.

Muscles have a vast capillary system. That's one reason why muscles use such a high level of nutrients to function. A pound of fat, by comparison, necessitates only 2 calories per day to exist. Muscle, therefore, is 18.75 times more active metabolically than the same amount of fat. The calorie-burning results of added muscle can have a positive, permanent effect on losing fat and keeping it off.

2. Muscle Moves Your Body

Muscle connects to tendons, and tendons cross joints and attach to bones. When muscles contract or shorten, they pull on bones, and the bones move. Movement of bones results in the flexion and extension of joints.

Although it may seem like an overly simple explanation of what happens to produce movement in your body, muscles are the only things that allow you to move. Hundreds of skeletal muscles can be contracted and relaxed to produce thousands and thousands of simple and complex actions.

Life as we know it is composed of movement. So if you want to improve your life, you must strengthen your ability to move. Proper exercise against resistance does that. It can make you a better word processor, piano player, walker, runner, swimmer, dancer, or singer. You name the action or activity, and proper exercise will help you do it better.

3. Muscle Strengthens Your Bones

Osteoporosis is a condition occurring mostly in women, in which bones become less dense, or more porous and brittle. Postmenopausal, small-boned, fair-complexioned, Caucasian women are in the high-risk group for osteoporosis. Bone thinning happens quietly without pain until one day a fracture or curvature of the spine becomes noticeable. Approximately half of the women who reach age 75 suffer at least one fracture due to osteoporosis.

Prevention and treatment of osteoporosis involves eating calcium-rich foods, taking calcium supplements, pursuing hormone therapy, and exercising. By far the most productive form of exercise for increasing bone density is strength training. Regularly stressing your muscles and bones against resistance encourages your body to lay down new bone cells. In fact, researchers at the University of Florida Center for Exercise Science recently verified this connection. They measured the bone-mineral density of 17 healthy volunteers between the ages of 62 and 82. These subjects were then placed on a once-a-week strength-training routine consisting of four exercises. After 6 months, they showed an average increase in bone-mineral density of 14 percent.

Because osteoporosis is such a debilitating disease, you should be doing muscle-building strength exercises even if you don't need to lose weight. It's that important.

Components of Body Weight

Do you weigh yourself on a bathroom scale every day? A lot of people do. Many believe it's an easy way to measure appearance and well-being. But it can be misleading. As I mentioned in Chapter 2, body weight is made up four components. They are:

- Bones

- Organs

- Muscles

- Fat

Your bones make up from 12 to 14 percent of your body weight, and your organs (including skin) occupy from 25 to 30 percent of it. Those items don't change significantly as you age. The remaining two, muscle and fat, do change. Much of the Tighten Your Tummy challenge centers on an understanding of muscle and fat—or, more specifically, optimizing your muscle-to-fat ratio.

The Average Woman

Over the past 30 years, I've done body composition measurements on more than 1,000 women. In addition, I've interviewed and observed the body shape problems of thousands more. The following chart describes the average body composition of the women (ages 14 to 50) whom I've trained and worked with as an exercise researcher.

My measurements and observations show that the average female's body contains the most muscle at age 14. At a height of 5 feet 5 inches and a body weight of 130 pounds, her muscle weighs 51 pounds and her fat weighs 24 pounds. Her muscle/fat ratio is 51/24 or 2.13/1. In other words, she has 2.13 pounds of muscle for each pound of fat. Because of this high ratio of muscle to fat, her body is firm, hard, and well defined.

With each passing year, however, she loses 0.5 pound of muscle and gains 1.5 pounds of fat if she does not do strength-training exercise. The specifics are listed in the chart.

Muscle/Fat Ratio Changes

Average Woman As She Ages

Age	14	20	30	40	50
Body weight (lbs)	130	136	146	156	166
Muscle (lbs)	51	48	43	38	33
Fat (lbs)	24	33	48	63	78
Percent body fat	18.5	24.3	32.9	40.4	47

From ages 14 to 50, women see their muscle mass decline and their fat increase.

At Age 50

At age 50, after birthing and raising an average of 2.2 children, the average American woman weighs 166 pounds, which is a gain of 36 pounds of body weight since age 14. More specifically, her muscle has decreased by 18 pounds and her fat has increased by 54 pounds. As a result, her percentage of body fat jumps from 18.5 to 47 percent—a 154 percent increase.

What causes this influx of fat and gradual loss of muscle? It's a combination of too many dietary calories, faulty eating habits, lack of proper exercise, pregnancy and childbirth, and the natural aging process.

More Muscle, Less Fat

To correct her figure problems, the average woman from her twenties to her fifties needs significantly less fat and more muscle. She needs what the Tighten Your Tummy program has to offer.

What about you? Are you similar to the average woman described in this chapter? Isn't it time you took action to improve your fat and muscle ratio?

You can't stop aging, but you can control every one of those other factors that lead to fat gain. With discipline, patience, and the guidelines presented in this book, you can successfully lose fat and build muscle at the same time. Doing so will have a significant effect on your muscle/fat ratio and an enormous effect on the appearance of your midsection, hips, thighs, and upper body.

Success stories of some of the women who have been through the program—including before-and-after photographs—appear throughout this book. Although each woman has unique physical characteristics, her body also resembles other female bodies in some respects. It will be useful for you to examine these photographs with an eye for figures similar to your own. Doing so will help you come to a realistic understanding of what you can achieve. And I believe you'll find it highly motivating.

You will also notice that none of the women pictured in this book has excessively large muscles or looks like a bodybuilder. But several of them have well-shaped body parts, which are shaped that way because of larger, stronger muscles. And get this: Several of these women want their muscles even larger.

For a woman to build excessively large muscles, she needs rare inherited characteristics. Such a woman would have to have unusually long muscle bellies and short tendons. This combination is even rare among men. Only one person in a million inherits these traits. Furthermore, to be a successful bodybuilder, a woman must be very lean. Once again, this necessitates favorable genetics, in that a person would have to have a well-below-average number of fat cells.

Larger muscles are in fact the very things women need. As I've stated earlier, adding muscle will help a woman to:

- Melt fat away

- Tighten flabby body parts

- Look better

- Improve movements throughout the body

- Strengthen bone

Don't be afraid of building excessively large muscles. It won't happen. If you ever did develop a muscle that was too large, all you'd have to do is stop exercising it. Within a week, the muscle would begin to atrophy, or lose size from disuse. Remember, a loss of muscle mass—at the rate of one-half pound per year—is the number-one fitness problem of most women.

Part II
THE SCIENCE OF FAT LOSS

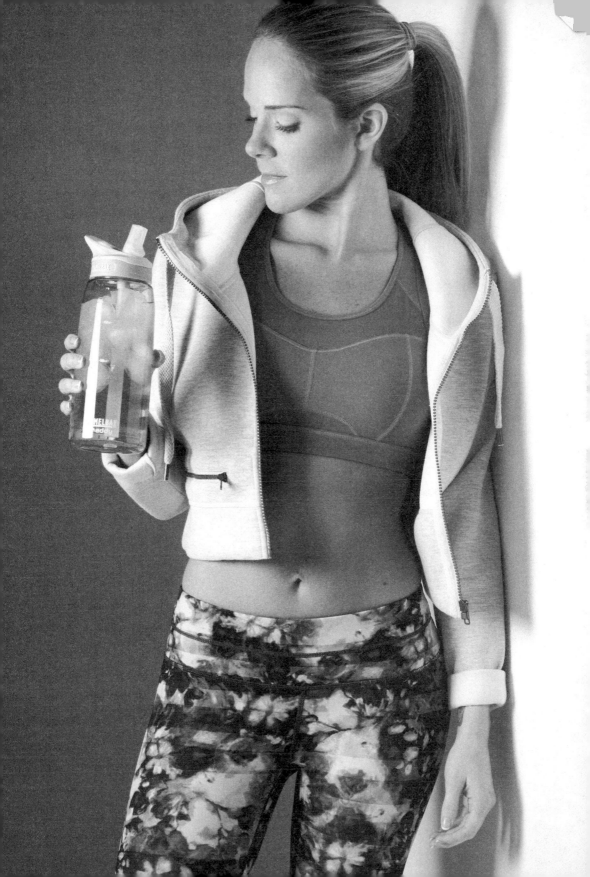

BEFORE & AFTER 6 WEEKS

Elena Mavrodieva
Age 40 • Height 5 feet, 8.5 inches

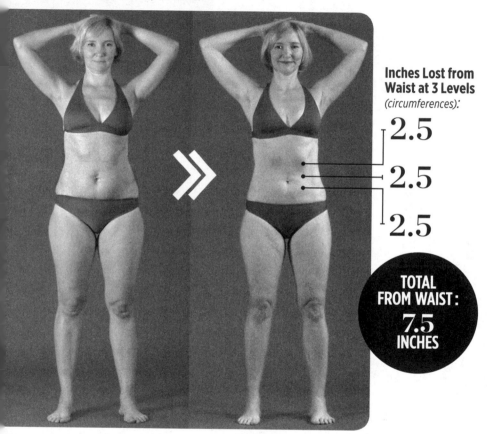

Inches Lost from Waist at 3 Levels *(circumferences):*

2.5

2.5

2.5

TOTAL FROM WAIST:
7.5 INCHES

Weight Before: **168.7 pounds**
Weight After: **153.5 pounds**
FAT LOSS: 18.76 pounds
Muscle Gain: **3.56 pounds**

"The extra muscle I gained really makes a difference in my daily life. I now feel stronger in just about everything I do."

—Elena Mavrodieva

chapter

4

A System for Shrinking Fat Cells

Understanding Your Anatomy and the Role of Hormones in Weight Loss

Part of conquering a bulging belly requires a basic understanding of what's going on below the surface of your midsection. You already know that your middle contains digestive organs, a backbone, and a few rolls of surface flab. But did you know that your waist also houses numerous hormone-secreting glands, eight major muscles, and billions of energy-storing cells? Being aware of the anatomy and the functions of these tissues will make a big difference in helping to tighten your tummy.

And did you know that your skin, that protective covering that stretches from head to belly to toe, is one of the most important factors in achieving a tighter tummy? You'll learn to apply a long-ignored function of this unique structure later in the book. For now, let's begin your anatomy lesson from the inside out.

Internal Organs

In the upper middle of your waist, tucked under your diaphragm, rest your stomach and liver. Slightly under those organs lie your pancreas and spleen. Below your stomach is the small intestine, which twists around in the center of your midsection at navel level and connects to the large intestine or colon. Your kidneys are housed here, too. Intersecting the bottom of your abdominal region is the pelvic cavity, which houses the internal reproductive organs, the urinary bladder, and the lower parts of the digestive system.

The midsection organs that are related to digestion are the stomach, liver, pancreas, small intestine, and large intestine. The spleen is an important organ in the lymphatic system. The two kidneys are the primary organs of the urinary system along with the bladder. The internal reproductive organs for the female are the ovaries, uterine tubes, and uterus.

This review may sound a bit like elementary school science, but what you may not have learned is that most of these organs contain glands that secrete hormones. Hormones are chemicals that stimulate, regulate, and inhibit various bodily processes and actions. As you'll see, certain hormones affect energy consumption, expenditure, and storage.

Influential Hormones

A number of hormones are key players in the Tighten Your Tummy program. Let's examine each one.

Insulin: The pancreas makes insulin. Its main function is to drive sugar and fat out of the bloodstream and into cells. The sugar can go into virtually any cell for use as fuel now or later. Most of the fat goes into your adipose tissues for storage.

Insulin is the most powerful pro-fat hormone and the primary promoter of fat preservation. The hormone is a holdover from the Ice Age, when it was an advantage to be able to quickly store as much fat as possible. Ample body fat meant survival when food was scarce. Insulin operates to conserve your fat stores by pushing your body to use sugar for energy instead of fat.

Big meals bring on big insulin responses, which tend to work against someone trying to lose fat. That's why you'll eat smaller meals on the Tighten Your Tummy plan. A meal of 300 calories or less brings on a small insulin response, meaning less fat storage.

Noradrenaline: This stimulant hormone is produced by your adrenal glands, which are near your kidneys. Noradrenaline causes your body to burn more calories, especially from fat cells.

The adrenal glands secrete noradrenaline under three conditions: cold temperature, hard exercise, and frequent eating. So you can influence the production of noradrenaline by keeping your body cool, performing high-intensity exercise, eating a small meal every 3 hours during the day, and sipping ice-cold water almost continuously throughout your waking hours.

Adrenaline: Also triggered by your adrenal glands, adrenaline mobilizes great surges of energy. It emerges when you're frightened or forced to respond quickly. Interestingly, adrenaline automatically speeds up your heart and respiration rates and extinguishes all desire to eat.

Estrogen: Estrogen is the best-known female hormone. At and after puberty, appropriate levels of estrogen cause fat to be deposited in the breasts, hips, and thighs of young girls. This powerful chemical influences the physiology of women in many ways throughout their lives. Estrogen is produced not only in the ovaries but also in the fat cells.

Progesterone: This is another female hormone that originates in the ovaries. Both progesterone and estrogen vary in somewhat of an inverse ratio during a normal menstrual cycle. During pregnancy, women have very high levels of progesterone and estrogen, which both accentuate fatness.

Progesterone is catabolic, which means it tends to break down muscle protein. Thus, when it is at its highest levels—usually a day or two before menstruation begins—most women feel sluggish and less motivated to exercise.

Serotonin: The nerves throughout your body secrete this well-publicized chemical. Research has established a strong relationship between serotonin and hunger. Low levels in the brain initiate hunger, and high levels curb hunger and make you feel full. Carbohydrate-rich foods do a good job of elevating serotonin. That's one reason why the Tighten Your Tummy diet provides 50 percent of its calories from carbohydrates.

Cholecystokinin: This interesting hormone is produced by your intestines mainly as fatty foods empty out of the stomach. Once cholecystokinin is secreted, it is picked up by the bloodstream, where it soon makes it way to the hypothalamus, or appetite-control center, in the brain. The end result is a feeling of fullness and satiety.

For any fat-loss diet to be most effective, it must supply a moderate amount of fatty foods daily. Such foods produce cholecystokinin, which in turn promotes satiety. That's why fats compose approximately 25 percent of the calories on the Tighten Your Tummy eating plan. You need fat to lose fat.

Ghrelin: Ghrelin is produced in your stomach, and it works with your brain to signal that you are hungry. Research shows that long after you have lost significant amounts of fat from your body, ghrelin doesn't forget—it wants you to regain the fat by constantly sending "hunger" signals to your brain. That's one reason why maintaining fat loss is often harder than losing it. Fortunately, you have a strategy for this, too: rigorous exercise. Intense exercise decreases ghrelin levels, making it a key component in fat-loss management.

Leptin: Leptin is a special hormone that is released from fat cells. It kicks in when your body starts losing fat by shutting down hunger and causing your body to mobilize and burn more fat as energy. You can maximize your body's leptin sensitivity by getting adequate sleep and rest.

Adiponectin: This is another chemical released by your fat cells. It boosts your metabolism, enhances your muscles' ability to use carbohydrates for energy, increases the rate at which your body breaks down fat, and curbs your appetite.

The Hormones of Muscle-Fat Cross Talk

In my 2014 book, *The Body Fat Breakthrough*, I reviewed more than 50 scientific studies and combined that information with my experiences and results at Gainesville Health & Fitness. I concluded that when negative-accentuated exercise impacts a person's level of strength by 30 to 50 percent, it also significantly affects at least six hormones this way:

- Stimulates growth hormone from the pituitary gland, which up-regulates the production of both insulin-like growth factor and mechano growth factor. Growth hormone also triggers the body to burn fat as fuel.

- Activates insulin-like growth factor, which is released by the liver and is important in muscle adaptation.

- Targets mechano growth factor, which kick-starts the muscle growth process.

- Mobilizes interleukin-6 within the muscle itself, where it merges into the blood to help overcompensate for inflammation from intense training.

- Triggers interleukin-15, which encourages cooperation between the processes of building muscle and metabolizing fat simultaneously.

- Directs the anabolic effects of insulin from the pancreas on both fat and muscle.

I suspect that negative-accentuated training brings into action a previously unknown hormone that unites these six hormones into a championship fat-burning team. This team can not only tighten your tummy but also turn your entire body into the lean, strong machine that it was originally designed to become.

Don't worry about understanding all of this. What you really need to believe is that the program of specialized exercise and diet in this book will influence these hormones, these chemical messengers, to enhance your body's ability to burn away the extra fat that is making your tummy flabby.

Muscles of the Midsection

Sheathing the internal organs on the front side of your waist are four layered muscles. Your lower and mid-back area contains your spine and four more major muscles. All of these muscles support and protect your internal organs, and they work to keep your pelvis and spine in proper alignment.

Let's take a look at each structure of what's generalized as "the abs."

Transverse abdominis: Of the four front muscles, this one lies innermost to your organs—until it crosses under your navel. When the lower fibers of this broad, flat, horizontal muscle get below the navel, they form a sheath opening with two other muscles. This permits the rectus abdominis to push through and attach securely to the pubic bone. As the transverse muscles contract, they compress the internal organs. This helps the lungs exhale and the body perform the normal process of elimination.

Internal oblique: This on-the-side muscle lies on top of the transverse abdominis. The muscle fibers start at the hip and run diagonally upward to meet the lower ribs. Lateral flexion and torso rotation to the same side are the main functions of the internal oblique muscles.

External oblique: This wide but thin muscle originates at the borders of the lower ribs and extends forward and downward. The fibers run at right angles to those of the internal oblique. The primary functions of the external oblique are to bend the spine to the same side and to rotate the torso to the opposite side.

Rectus abdominis: The outermost frontal muscle stretches vertically from the rib cage to the pubic bone. The function of the rectus abdominis is to shorten the distance between the breastbone and the pelvic girdle. A lean woman with well-developed rectus abdominis on each side of the midline can usually display three paired blocks of muscle. These blocks are caused by crossing tendinous inscriptions.

Psoas major, quadratus lumborum, erector spinae, and latissimus dorsi: These four muscles attach to, move, or support your lumbar spine. When the muscles of your lower back are strong, they create a tight protective girdle around your spine. Weak lower-back muscles—combined with weak abdominal and oblique muscles—encourage the spine to sag toward the front of the body, which may lead to injury and pain. Strong lower-back, abdominal, and oblique muscles help you to maintain a healthy, upright posture, which allows you to look better, feel better, and perform better in sports and recreational activities.

Fat Cells

Intermingled in and around the muscles and organs of your midsection is a yellowish-white tissue called fat. At body temperature, fat is a thick liquid. It feels semisolid in your bulges because the walls of the fat cell keep it in place.

Seen under a microscope, fat cells look like a bubble bath. The globules are grouped together with stringy intercellular glue and streaked with narrow filaments of connective tissue, blood vessels, and nerves. The network of fat cells forms a versatile living inner tube, for the cells can inflate or deflate as required.

Throughout your midsection you have billions of fat cells. That's right, billions with a *b*. In fact, scientists have taken samples from throughout the human body and actually counted the number of cells. Although this research depends on extrapolation, some interesting findings emerge.

- The number of fat cells can vary greatly from person to person, depending primarily on genetic factors. Numbers range from a low of 10 billion to a high of 250 billion. Obviously, a person with a minimum number of fat cells has a lower probability of being obese compared to a person with a high number of fat cells.

- Research reveals that the average woman in the United States has approximately 42 billion fat cells. The average man has fewer, about 25 billion fat cells.

- Body fat is composed of 79 percent lipids, 15 percent water, and 6 percent proteins. It is because of the high concentration of lipids that fat contains so many calories. The 3,500 calories in a pound of fat is almost six times the number of calories in the same amount of muscle tissue.

- Fat is your most concentrated way of storing the fuel it needs for energy. Fat also provides insulation, warmth, and protection to your muscles and internal organs. Without such warmth, even a light breeze would send you scurrying for a coat.

- Fat is crucial for reproduction, which is why women average 68 percent more fat cells than men. Also many female hormones, as discussed earlier, share regulatory relationships with fat cells.

Even if you are not blessed with the best genetics—which means that you may have several times as many fat cells as the average woman—you can successfully shrink your fat cells. You can still lose significant pounds and inches from your waist and elsewhere.

Skin Facts

Few people realize that the skin is the body's largest organ. Surprisingly, an average woman's skin would cover approximately 20 square feet if it were laid out flat. This overall size, or surface area, is the primary reason why as much as 85 percent of the heat you transmit each day emerges through your skin. And heat loss, in case you didn't know it, is directly related to fat loss.

It's important that you understand the following connection: Fat throughout your body is energy. Energy is best expressed as calories, which are units of heat measurement. One ounce of body fat supplies 219 calories, and 1 pound contains approximately 3,500 calories.

Your body uses hundreds of calories each day to keep it functioning. These calories are generated from the foods you consume and from energy storage spots, such as fat cells around your waist. Although your body resorts to several different energy-producing pathways, all of them require calories. Calories count significantly in the fat-loss equation.

Heat calories transfer out of your skin by radiation, conduction, convection, and evaporation. Approximately 50 percent of the calories eliminated through your skin each day are lost as radiant heat. Radiation is why a tall woman has an easier time losing fat than a shorter woman of the same weight. A taller woman has more skin available to the environment than a shorter woman and thus is able to radiate more heat.

Conduction is the transfer of calories through direct contact. For example, when you get into a cool swimming pool, heat from your body immediately goes into the water. Water is a much better conductor than air, so you can lose more calories in cold water than in cold air. Drinking chilled water is another way to take advantage of conduction, which I'll discuss in Chapter 8. To be almost shivering, which is another example of conduction, also stimulates your adrenal glands to produce noradrenaline—which in turn causes your body to burn more calories.

Your skin disposes of another 15 percent of heat by convection. This means that air is circulating around your skin to move away the heat. That's why the wind makes you feel cooler when you bicycle or walk. That's why an overhead fan in a workout room can benefit the heat-loss process as you exercise below.

While you may not be aware of it, your skin perspires constantly. This unnoticeable perspiration is eliminated by evaporation. At ordinary room temperatures, the moisture vaporized from your skin, plus that from your lungs, accounts for approximately 25 percent of the calories lost from your body at rest. One-third of the heat loss by evaporation is removed through your lungs and the other two-thirds from invisible perspiration on your skin.

Few people have ever considered the impact that keeping the skin cool has on the fat-loss process. When I started incorporating this concept into my standard diet and exercise routine for test groups in 1990, I immediately noticed a significant improvement in the average fat loss among these groups compared to previous groups that did not use this technique. Since then, I've continually refined the keeping-cool concept, and I'll cover it in Chapter 19.

Interrelationships and the Program

You should now begin to realize how closely your internal organs, hormones, muscles, fat cells, and skin work together. Can you see how simply cutting back on your eating and increasing your exercising is not enough, especially if you are serious about getting rid of your tummy fast? You need to be strategic about your diet and your exercise routine in order to trigger your hormones to influence your muscles and fat cells. The composition of your calories and the way you perform exercises play key roles in how effectively all of your internal systems work together to use energy. Plus, let's not forget how important your skin is in facilitating heat loss (i.e., fat loss). You'll maximize that effect by keeping cool and drinking plenty of cold water. Tighten Your Tummy in 2 Weeks incorporates all of these interrelationships into result-producing actions.

It is important to understand that the living inner tube of fatty cells that surrounds your waist contains too much liquid fat. Your goal is to deflate your inner tube—in the fastest way possible.

To accomplish this goal, you must send the correct messages to your system to give up the calories within your fat cells and transfer them out of your body. For more than four decades, I've researched the most effective ways to cause these complicated interrelationships within your body to maximize fat loss. And I've incorporated them into a simple program of steps you will take every day—a smart eating plan, a negative-accentuated exercising routine, a productive resting schedule, and a powerful superhydrating system—to help you eliminate excess body fat.

Soon your body will be lean and your belly will be tight.

BEFORE & AFTER 2 WEEKS

Kristi Taylor

Age 39 • Height 5 feet, 7.5 inches

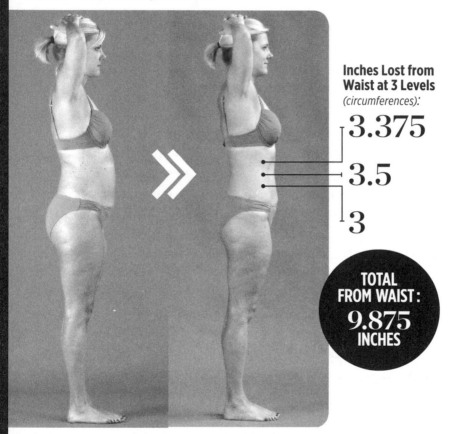

**Inches Lost from
Waist at 3 Levels**
(circumferences):

3.375
3.5
3

**TOTAL
FROM WAIST:
9.875
INCHES**

Weight Before: **150.8 pounds**
Weight After: **141.9 pounds**
FAT LOSS: 11.4 pounds
Muscle Gain: **2.5 pounds**

"For the first time, an
exercise program has
made a real difference.
And in just 2 weeks!"

—Kristi Taylor

chapter

5

The Training Technique for a Tighter Tummy

The Science behind the Method

Your midsection is made up of various muscles that have the ability to contract or shorten and hold and support. But these muscles can also lengthen, stretch, and relax.

Physiologists have named the contraction process *concentric muscle action*. The opposite of contraction is lengthening, which is called *eccentric muscle action*. *Concentric* means moving toward the center of the body, and *eccentric* means moving away from the center.

Let's take the simple situp with bent knees to illustrate both actions. From a lying position, the sitting-up movement involves concentric action of the abdominal muscles. Returning to the lying position requires eccentric muscle action. It's a simple concept that is very important to this book.

Bodybuilders, weight lifters, and strength coaches use the words *positive* to mean concentric muscle action and *negative* to mean eccentric muscle action. In bodybuilding circles, lifting a weight is positive and lowering is negative. The same is true when using a weight machine. As the weight stack moves up, positive work is being done. As it moves down, negative work is accomplished. For ease of understanding, I'll use the words *positive* and *negative,* instead of *concentric* and *eccentric,* in this book.

For more than 60 years, researchers have compared the various aspects of positive and negative training. In 1953, Erling Asmussen, PhD, an exercise physiologist at the University of Copenhagen, Denmark, was the first to point out in a scientific journal the differences between positive and negative actions on muscles. The measuring tools and techniques he applied were crude. Decades later, in the 1980s, my colleague Arthur Jones of Nautilus Sports/Medical Industries developed tools and methods that made testing the positive and negative movements easier to repeat and, as a result, more valid.

Jones discovered that both women and men were approximately 40 percent stronger while doing the negative portion of a lift on an exercise machine, compared to the positive stroke. He surmised that if one could add more resistance to the negative phase versus the positive, one could build stronger muscle faster. Jones eventually developed fitness machines that allowed the weight being moved to change during the course of one repetition, making it more efficient and effective. The secret was in the shape of the cam or gear on the machine, which resembled a nautilus shell. He developed exercise machines based on this design, and Nautilus was born. The machines, which appeared in health clubs throughout the world, revolutionized the fitness industry.

Athletes and fitness-minded people devoured Jones's research and began applying negative work in their weekly strength-training programs. Negative training became a hot topic, and the more the scientific journals and muscle and fitness magazines reported, the more misunderstanding grew. Additional research on negative training over the next 20 years and the reported results were inconsistent, causing many to doubt the benefits of negative training.

Meta-Analysis and Negative Training

When Marc Roig, PhD, was the head of the Muscle Biophysics Laboratory at the University of British Columbia in Vancouver, he and his colleagues saw the disparities in the published research and decided to sort things out by using newer types of statistical tests called meta-analysis. Meta-analysis comprises statistical methods for contrasting and combining findings from different reports in the quest to identify patterns among study results.

Dr. Roig's group carefully examined all the published studies over the last 50 years that compared negative-style resistance training with normal positive training. At first, they identified 1,954 titles from their literature search. Of this number, 276 were suitable for abstract review. More than 60 publications made the next cut. Deeper examinations narrowed the studies down to exactly 20.

These 20 studies involved a total of 678 subjects, and in the studies that provided gender, 58 percent of the trainees were females. The usual training frequency was three times per week, and the duration of the experiments ranged from 4 to 25 weeks, with the most popular duration being 6 weeks. Dr. Roig and his researchers entered all the data from those studies to create computerized meta-analyses. The results, published in the *British Journal of Sports Medicine* (2009), showed that "negative training was significantly more effective in increasing muscular size and strength than positive-style training."

I remember reading Dr. Roig's report with much interest. Not only had I been interested in negative training for more than 20 years, I also had been contacted a year earlier by another pioneer of negative training, Mats Thulin of Stockholm, Sweden. Thulin told me that he had designed a new type of exercise machine that "accentuated the negative" to a greater degree than even Arthur Jones's Nautilus.

The X-Force

I flew to Stockholm on November 13, 2008, to meet with Thulin and try out his new negative-accentuated equipment. He called his machines X-Force, and they operated differently than any other exercise equipment I'd ever seen.

Thulin's workout machines have a tilting weight stack powered by an electric servomotor. As the user begins the positive stroke, the weight stack sits at a 45-degree angle. This angle reduces the selected resistance significantly. Then, at the top of the positive stroke, the tilted weight stack moves to a vertical position, which causes the resistance to become instantly 40 percent heavier. The user then lowers 100 percent of the selected resistance.

After training with X-Force machines for 3 days and exploring the physiology with Thulin and his team, I was convinced of its overall potential. The ingenuity of the X-Force equipment is a patented, tilting weight stack that unloads the positive phase and then overloads the negative. X-Force

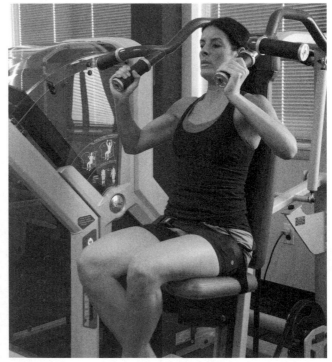

This is the X-Force Deltoid Press machine in use. The plastic-encased assembly on the left side of the photo houses the weight stack, which tilts 45 degrees, providing less resistance for the positive phase of the lift. Once the trainee straightens her arms, the weight stack will tilt back to the vertical, which automatically makes the resistance 40 percent heavier on the lowering, or negative, portion of the lift.

equipment—a total of 14 strength-training machines—supplies negative-accentuated exercise, 40 percent more negative resistance compared to the positive.

When I returned to the United States, I knew I had to get the X-Force line installed near my home in Florida, so I could continue my research into better ways to lose fat and build muscle. One of the first people I talked with about this was Joe Cirulli of Gainesville Health & Fitness. Cirulli had always wanted to pursue various fat-loss and muscle-building projects with me, and X-Force was no exception.

It took a lot of discussion and planning, but in January 2012, Cirulli's fitness center was outfitted with 14 X-Force machines. Gainesville and Orlando, near my home, are an easy drive from each other, so I knew I could quickly get a research project together. The next month, I started my first of multiple test groups training on X-Force equipment. By December 2012, I had trained eight groups on X-Force, with a total of 145 participants from the fitness center. And those groups achieved remarkable results.

Unfortunately, X-Force machines are very expensive and hard to find. At the time, only a handful of fitness clubs in the United States owned them. To help other people achieve the kind of results my X-Force test panelists achieved, I knew I had to find an alternative method for those without access to these high-tech tools. That's how I developed the 30-30-30 negative-accentuated training method that formed the backbone of my book *The Body Fat Breakthrough: Tap the Muscle-Building Power of Negative Training and Lose up to 30 Pounds in 30 Days.*

30-30-30

Through trial-and-error testing, I found that performing $1\frac{1}{2}$ repetitions of an exercise extremely slowly—30 seconds on the negative, 30 seconds on the positive, and another 30-second negative—proved to be the best alternative to X-Force.

To perform 30-30-30 properly, you'll start by preparing a barbell or weight machine using 80 percent of the weight or resistance you'd normally handle for 10 repetitions. Have an assistant help you get the weight to the top position. Then do a slow 30-second negative, followed by a 30-second positive, followed by a final 30-second negative. That's 1½ repetitions, or 60 seconds of negative work and 30 seconds of positive work. That's one set, and that's all you need to do for each of six exercises. The exercises I selected from were the leg press, leg curl, leg extension, chest press, pulldown to chest, overhead press, curl, and abdominal crunch. The 30-30-30 system proved to be an excellent way to build strength and burn fat.

After the publication of *Body Fat Breakthrough,* I began experimenting with variations of this extra slow exercise method. Could I discover a workout that was less intense yet equally effective? After a couple of months of experimentation, I developed something even more useful and easier, especially for women.

15-15-15

Essentially, it's just a shorter version of 30-30-30. Instead of taking 30 seconds to perform each half of 1½ repetitions, I've shortened each phase to 15 seconds. Here's how you do it:

Again, set up free weights or a weight machine using 80 percent of the weight or resistance you'd normally handle. Get the resistance to the top position quickly, then do the first negative phase slowly, taking 15 seconds, followed by a 15-second positive and another 15-second negative. But don't stop. Without resting, do a series of faster, complete repetitions to a count of approximately 1 second on the positive and 2 seconds on the negative. Your goal is to complete 8 to 12 of the faster repetitions. And again, only one set of each exercise is necessary. I found that doing six to eight exercises this way twice a week is all that's needed for remarkable results when teamed with the four other parts of the Tighten Your Tummy program.

That's it. An exercise session of 15-15-15, plus 8 to 12 repetitions, takes no more than 30 minutes. I supervised two test-panel groups during the fall of 2014, and both responded well. How does it work? Well, the three very slow half reps thoroughly fatigue the involved muscles; following that with 8 to 12 regular repetitions causes an intense "burn" in those fatigued muscles. I believe that a short but slow single bout of weight-bearing exercises causes deeper inroad in your muscles, triggering the release of multiple hormones that burn calories from surrounding fat cells.

The technique worked superbly on short-range abdominal floor exercises, body-weight movements such as the squat and pushup, and dumbbell exercises such as the curl and overhead press. I think this negative-accentuated 15-15-15 technique is the best way to flatten your belly fast, which is why it's the cornerstone of the Tighten Your Tummy program. In summary, my new 15-15-15 plus 8 to 12 repetitions concept does not require elaborate machines. It works great on just about any freehand floor exercise or movements performed with barbells and dumbbells. Chapter 10 provides a complete discussion of the specific exercises that I recommend.

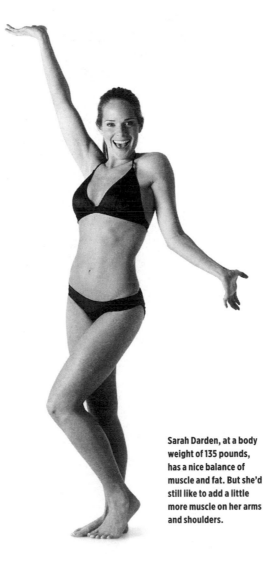

Sarah Darden, at a body weight of 135 pounds, has a nice balance of muscle and fat. But she'd still like to add a little more muscle on her arms and shoulders.

BEFORE & AFTER 2 WEEKS

Denise Rodriguez
Age 34 • Height 5 feet, 7.75 inches

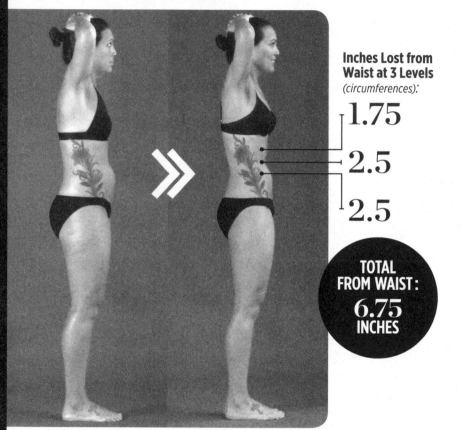

Inches Lost from Waist at 3 Levels
(circumferences):

1.75

2.5

2.5

TOTAL FROM WAIST:
6.75
INCHES

Weight Before: **155.7 pounds**

Weight After: **143.6 pounds**

FAT LOSS: 14.49 pounds

Muscle Gain: **2.1 pounds**

"For the longest time, I wouldn't dare eat much in the way of carbs. Now, I'm not afraid to consume them—lots of them!"

—Denise Rodriguez

chapter

6

Nutrition for Fat Loss

Welcome Back Carbohydrates!

Diets don't work.

Google that phrase and you'll get more than 41 million references. Generally, if you peruse the first dozen or so of these articles, you'll read this: Most diets seem to succeed in the short term and fail in the long term.

You've probably heard that before. In all likelihood, you've experienced it firsthand a number of times. Yet I'm here to tell you that *diets do work*—if, and that's a big IF—they are grounded in certain fundamental principles of nutrition.

What are those fundamentals? They are the basics taught in major university nutrition departments throughout the United States. You'll find them in every textbook for introductory nutrition courses. The problem is that most of those aren't very exciting to read. Some students might even say they are boring. Compared to a lot of the best-selling diet books, which are often based on nothing more than sensational promises, these nutrition manuals don't get much attention.

In this chapter, we'll explore some of the key science-backed nutrition concepts found in those books, but this won't be a comprehensive view of basic nutrition. It would take far too many pages to do that. If you are interested, however, here are two introductory texts on nutrition that I really like—and they are not boring. Just the opposite: Both are well-written and beautifully illustrated.

- *Nutrition: Concepts and Controversies* (paperback, 13th edition), by Frances Sizer and Ellie Whitney, Wadsworth Cengage Learning, 2013

- *Understanding Nutrition* (hardcover, 14th edition), by Ellie Whitney and Sharon Rady Rolfes, Cengage Learning, 2014

Both books are published in multiple formats and can be expensive, if purchased new. Their previous editions, however, can be purchased on Amazon.com at bargain prices.

Criteria for a Safe, Effective Diet

Do you know how many weight-loss diets are available in the United States? Check Amazon or go into a bookstore, and you'll get a sense that the number must be staggering. And each year, more diet books and Internet weight-loss programs are introduced. Some years ago, researchers with the Health, Weight, and Stress program at Johns Hopkins University discovered 29,000 different methods for losing weight. They collected and analyzed them, and found that less than 6 percent were effective or even safe. So how can an average consumer be expected to know whether a diet works or if it is dangerous?

Let me tell you a story: When I was in graduate school at Florida State University (1968–1973), my first home was the exercise-science department. But my second home was the nutrition department. In fact, I completed 2 years of postdoctoral study with Dr. Harold E. Schendel, a professor of nutrition. Sharing the office with him for several years was a young woman who had just completed her doctorate at Washington University in St. Louis. Her name was Eleanor Whitney.

Dr. Whitney had a great love for research and writing. I learned a lot from her, and we often talked about the challenges of making the basics of good nutrition more available to the general population. Throughout her career, she has done a great job of making detailed research meaningful and applicable to the average reader through her books and textbooks. And through her research, Dr. Whitney developed a very useful list of seven criteria for a safe, effective diet. In question form, they are as follows:

- Does the diet provide a reasonable number of calories—an absolute minimum of 1,000 calories a day?

- Does it supply enough but not too much protein—at least the recommended 0.4 gram per pound of body weight but not more than twice that much?

- Does it supply enough fat for satiety but not too much—so that between 20 and 35 percent of the day's total calories come from fat?

- Does it supply enough carbohydrate to spare protein, so that you won't burn muscle tissue for energy and won't prevent the liver from running out of glycogen (ketosis)—about 100 grams of carbohydrate for the average-size person?

- Does it provide a balanced assortment of vitamins and minerals from whole food sources in all of the basic food groups?

- Does it offer different foods every day so that you won't give up on the diet out of boredom?

- Does it consist of ordinary foods that are available in supermarkets at prices you can afford?

No matter which diet you try, make sure it meets those criteria. Lucky for you, the Tighten Your Tummy diet answers yes to all of her questions.

Dieting Doesn't Have to Be Difficult

When I wrote *The Nautilus Diet* in 1987, I included 72 recipes, many of which required more than an hour of preparation and cooking time. In my 2014 diet program, *The Body Fat Breakthrough*, I have only seven recipes and two of them relate to salads, which require no more than 5 minutes to prepare.

Today convenience, speed, and simplicity are priorities. Fortunately, my research has uncovered some interesting eating behaviors that prove dieting doesn't have to be complicated. Here are some of my observations:

- Dieters can eat the same breakfast each day for 6 weeks or more.

- Dieters can eat the same lunch each day for 6 weeks. After 6 weeks, they like a second choice for lunch.

- Approximately 75 percent of dieters can adapt to a meal-replacement shake mix for breakfast or lunch.

- Dieters like variety for dinner. Typically, they like to have three meal options from which to choose.

- Approximately 70 percent of dieters find that the convenience and built-in portion control of frozen microwave dinners help them stick to their diets.

- Dieters like in-between-meal snacks.

Keeping these observations in mind, let's take a look at some other key parts of the weight-loss equation: meal composition, meal size, meal frequency, and calories per day.

Meal Composition

A recent dietary survey found that the typical U.S. adult gets 46 percent of her or his daily calories from carbohydrates, 37 percent from fats, and 17 percent from proteins. Despite the popularity of paleo-style diets, most nutritional scientists agree that Americans would be better off with more carbohydrates and less fats.

The majority of nutritional scientists also believe that carbohydrate-rich foods should make up at least 50 percent of a dieter's meals. I concur. In fact, after working with thousands of men and women who wanted to reduce fat, I've found that what works best is consuming about 50 percent carbohydrates, 25 percent fats, and 25 percent proteins every day.

A 50:25:25 breakdown for each meal influences certain hormones, such as serotonin and cholecystokinin, which are important in producing satiation, the process of feeling full and satisfied.

Meal Size

Consuming small meals will help you lose weight. But there's a thin line between a small meal and a medium meal, which makes a big difference. I draw the line at 300 calories for women and 400 calories for men.

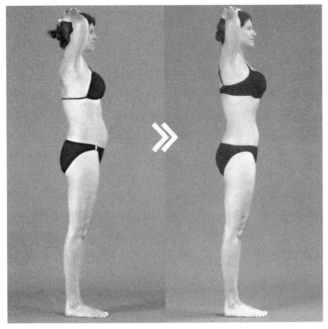

Six-foot-tall Barbara Trombetta lost 12.43 pounds of fat during the first 2 weeks of the TYT test panel program. She was amazed that she could eat a carbohydrate-rich diet and still become leaner.

Small meals facilitate fat loss because they trigger tiny insulin responses. Insulin, a hormone produced in your pancreas, is the most powerful pro-fat hormone and the primary promoter of fat preservation. It's a holdover from the Ice Age, when it was to a human's advantage to be able to quickly store as much fat as possible. Ample body fat meant survival when food was scarce.

Thus, the meals and snacks that I recommend for fat loss are always 300 calories or fewer for women.

Small meals will help you to:

- Prevent mood changes caused by low blood sugar

- Temper food cravings caused by low blood sugar

- Reduce PMS and menopausal tension

- Eliminate the starvation response elicited by skipping meals

- Lose fat because you'll never be putting your body in the storage mode

- Experience more energy in all that you do—including your negative-accentuated training program

Meal Frequency

The goal for the Tighten Your Tummy program is five or six small, evenly spaced meals a day. This means that no longer than 3 hours should elapse between eating something. You'll have breakfast, lunch, and dinner, and snacks at midmorning, midafternoon, and night. In this book, a snack of 50 to 100 calories is considered a small meal. The sum of the five or six small meals, or the total number of calories that you consume each day, is the remaining key factor.

Calories Per Day

Remember that 1 gram of carbohydrate and 1 gram of protein each supply 4 calories, while 1 gram of fat contains 9 calories. All calories from those macronutrients count in losing body fat. The key to losing fat and weight is consuming fewer calories than you burn. However, your reduction in calories should not be so low that your body pulls nutrients from your muscles and vital organs. That's counterproductive.

The majority of the dieters I've worked with achieve optimum results by adhering to daily calorie levels that range from 1,000 to 1,500. Women respond best to 1,000 to 1,300 calories a day. Men require slightly more, approximately 1,200 to 1,500 per day. This keeps your body well fueled so that your muscle isn't compromised. You lose fat rather than lean muscle. A slight variation in the total number of daily calories on a weekly basis is also helpful.

Learn to Love "Hydrated Carbons"

You're probably wondering about the high-carb emphasis in the program's eating plan. After all, so much has been made in the press about the so-called dangers of carbohydrates and benefits of high-protein diets. Let me address those concerns with a little story of Terrie Baker, 44, a tall, attractive mother of two children who used to live down the street from me. I would frequently talk with her at the bus stop as we waited for our kids to arrive back from school. Terrie was a chronic dieter. She was skinny but still had excessive fat around her waist and hips. And she always wanted to look like what she called "California cut." In her quest for leanness, she focused on protein foods and avoided carbs. She had practiced a strict Atkins eating plan on and off for many years. Curious about my work, she often asked me about my training programs in Gainesville.

When I finished my research for *The Body Fat Breakthrough* in 2013, I assembled about 25 of my best before-and-after photos and placed them in an organized manner in a folder. The next day, I invited Terrie over to my home gym to look through the pictures. She was impressed and wanted to know what kind of diet these subjects were on.

Here was my dilemma. I wanted to help Terrie, but I knew if I told her that these people consumed a carbohydrate-rich diet, she'd either dismiss it as malarkey or ask me for a detailed explanation, which I didn't have the time to do. I also knew she had been a critical care nurse at one time. So I threw her a quick-breaking curve ball.

"At least 50 percent of these dieters' calories came from hydrated carbons," I said. "That's the primary reason their muscles are so solid, tight looking, and cut." (I made sure to get the word *cut* in there.) I could see her mind working overtime with the concept of *hydrated carbons*. I went to the part of my library that contained my biochemistry texts and pulled out one that showed the molecular structure of both simple and complex hydrated carbons, more commonly called carbohydrates. I opened the book wide on my desk and showed her the array of carbon (C), hydrogen (H), and oxygen (O) atoms and how they interplayed and hooked together to form mono-, di-, and polysaccharides.

Then I said, "These different compounds, or hydrated carbons, inside the human body give your muscles and organs the ability to store water in large amounts."

I waited for her to take the words *hydrated carbon* and turn them around in her mind and get . . . *carbo-hydrate.*

After at least 10 seconds, it suddenly hit her. "OMG," she said. "Where have I been for the last 5 years? I've got to rework my thinking and eating . . . and . . . learn to love hydrated carbons."

Shortly thereafter, Terrie's husband got a business offer in California, and the family moved to San Diego. And Terrie started on a new eating plan, getting 50 percent of her calories from quality, carbohydrate-rich foods. She now loves her "hydrated carbons," and as a result, she is stronger, leaner, and more "California cut" than ever before.

Remember: Carbohydrates ("hydrated carbons") are the ideal nutrients to meet your body's energy needs, keep your digestive system fit, feed your brain and nervous system, and support body leanness.

BEFORE & AFTER 6 WEEKS

Melissa Jones
Age 36 • Height 5 feet, 6 inches

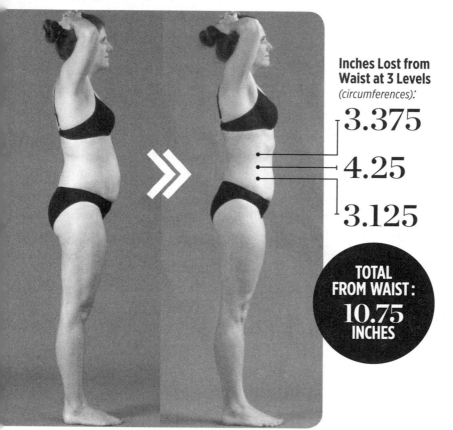

Inches Lost from Waist at 3 Levels
(circumferences):

3.375

4.25

3.125

TOTAL FROM WAIST:
10.75
INCHES

Weight Before: **154.5 pounds**
Weight After: **142.7 pounds**
FAT LOSS: 19.49 pounds
Muscle Gain: **7.69 pounds**

"Everyone at work asked about my weight loss, but it was my husband who noticed more than anyone."
—*Melissa Jones*

chapter

7

How Hydration Fuels Fat Loss

Drink More Water, Weigh Less

The fountain of youth is just a sip away. It's free, refreshing, and comes with a 100 percent guarantee to make you feel great.

Here's the case for superhydration. Up to 75 percent of your muscle mass is composed of water. That's why good hydration is so essential for an exercise program. It gives your muscles their natural ability to expand and contract during workouts. Water also helps hydrate your skin to prevent the sagging that can accompany weight loss. When your fat cells shrink, the skin can get wrinkly. Water plumps the skin, leaving it clear, healthy, and resilient.

Water is critical for the proper functioning of your organs. If you don't drink enough water every day, your body's reaction is to retain what water it does have. This causes waste products to accumulate and hamper kidney function. When that happens, your body sends a signal to your liver to come to the rescue to flush out the impurities. That's a lifesaver, but it comes at a price: It takes your liver away from one of its key functions: metabolizing stored body fat into usable energy. As a result, fat buildup occurs, and your body weight increases. Do you see how something as innocent as being a little dehydrated can create such a damaging domino effect?

Your Weapon against Weight: A Water Bottle

Even though I don't know you, I can make a pretty accurate guess that you are chronically dehydrated. Consider this: It's estimated that 41 percent of women do not drink the recommended eight 8-ounce glasses of water every day. That's what the government recommends, and yet for people who do intense exercise or want to lose fat, 64 ounces is not nearly enough. That's why on the Tighten Your Tummy plan, I recommend that you consume 16 glasses of water (that's a gallon, 128 ounces) every day.

I'm not saying it's supereasy to do, but it's easier than you think, as my test panelists found out. Invest in a 32-ounce tumbler—preferably one that's insulated and has a built-in straw. Keep it in tow throughout the day and night, and drink up! Refill it four times. You'll be surprised how quickly you will adapt to this routine.

To turbocharge your fat loss, the water you drink should be ice-cold. In my previous books, I recommended drinking water that's 40 degrees Fahrenheit because it takes 123 calories of body heat to warm the 128 ounces to your core body temperature of 98.6 degrees. But for Tighten Your Tummy, I want your water to be about 32 degrees Fahrenheit. For years, I've been underestimating the calorie-burning power of ice-cold water. Not anymore. The chilly temperature will tap your body's metabolism to burn an extra 140 calories to maintain your core temperature.

THE ICE-WATER DIET
DRINKING 1 GALLON OF ICE WATER burns an additional 140 calories per day.

Feeling Fuller and Other Benefits

You are what you drink. Top off your tank with water, and forget snacking or overindulging at dinner.

Water can also keep you from overeating by inflating your belly, which signals your brain that you are satisfied and not hungry. And it ensures that you're filling up with zero calories, not sugary beverages high in empty calories. Drink two glasses of water before every meal and snack. Help your satiety last even longer by eating high-fiber foods, which will absorb the water and swell in size.

Drinking a gallon of water a day has another slimming effect: The more you drink, the more you go—to the ladies' room, that is. Remember in Chapter 4, when I noted sources of heat loss from your body? Fat is transferred out of the body in the form of heat through your skin. Heat, calories, and fat are also eliminated as you pass urine. As a bonus, more frequent bathroom breaks means more calories being burned from extra walking, especially when the restroom is on the second floor! Another bonus: greater regularity. If you don't drink enough water, your body pulls it from your lower intestine, creating hard, drier stools. But drink a gallon of water a day and you won't suffer from constipation.

The Only Drink You'll Ever Need

Water is the diamond of beverages—it's clear, pure, and the most valuable one you can buy. Every other beverage pales in comparison like a cheap cubic zirconia.

There is a difference between water and other beverages that contain water. Biochemically they may look the same, but as with diamonds and cubic zirconias, there's definitely a difference in quality. While you can

WHAT YOU CAN LEARN FROM A CLUCKING CHICKEN

IN AT LEAST ONE WAY, CHICKENS are smarter than humans. A laying hen can sense when she's becoming dehydrated, and she'll let a farmer know by clucking loudly in a very recognizable "squeaky squawk." Hens instinctively know the importance of lots of fresh water for egg laying. And so do egg farmers, who have a financial stake in keeping their "workers" in close proximity to fresh water. They know that denying a laying hen water for 24 hours will make that chicken's egg production drop 40 percent. Go 48 hours without supplying water and they'll never get another egg from that hen.

What do chickens have to do with women? Well, chickens' bodies are made up of muscle, fat, organs, and bones just as ours are. Consider what happens when you withhold water from a hen. You get rapid atrophy of the muscles and organs, which is why egg production grinds to a halt. What's more, as the hen's muscles shrink, her percentage of body fat increases proportionately. The same thing can happen in your body, much more slowly for sure, but the chicken example shows how essential proper hydration is to good health and reducing body fat.

still consume the ounces of H_2O you need every day from other beverages such as soft drinks, tea, coffee, beer, fruit-flavored punches, and all-natural fruit juices such as orange juice and apple cider, these liquids also contain substances that contradict water's positive effects.

Soft drinks, tea, and coffee can contain caffeine, which stimulates the adrenal glands and acts as a diuretic. So as you run to the bathroom with a pounding headache, you'll still be thirsty. When you're dehydrated, you may experience headaches, fatigue, worsened mood, and difficulty concentrating.

Other beverages—like juice, alcohol, and, again, soda—are loaded with sugar and calories. Flavored drinks can actually create a distaste for pure water. You can become so reliant on the sweet flavor that plain water becomes unappealing. So stick with a classic: tap water. And unless you're taking a trip to a questionable country, tap water is as good as or even safer than bottled. And a lot cheaper. Going abroad? Bottled water is great on the go.

A Salient Note

You can have too much of a good thing. Although rare, water intoxication—drinking too much water—can cause you to become sick. And a few ailments can be negatively affected by drinking large amounts of fluids. To be safe, check with your physician before consuming the gallon of ice water daily that I'm recommending.

Part III
BEST TUMMY TIGHTENERS

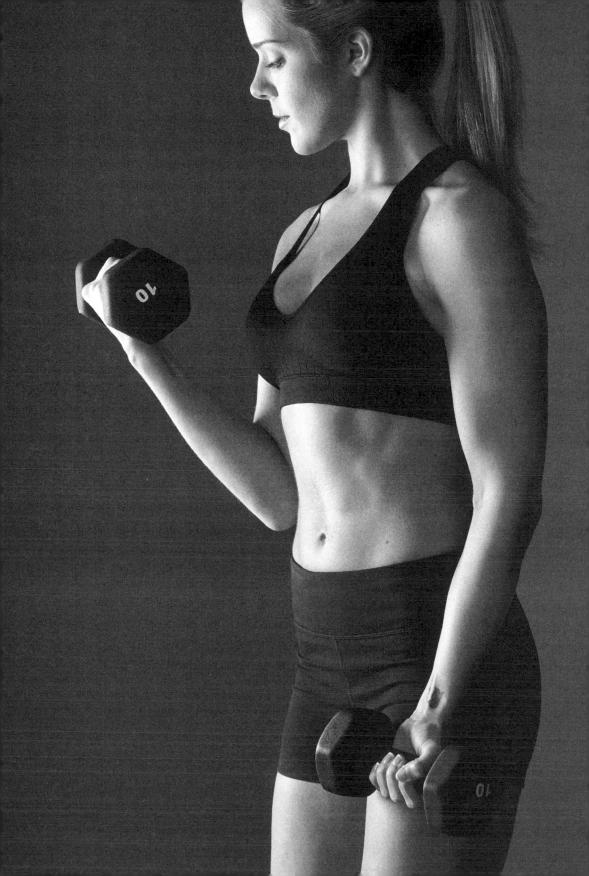

BEFORE & AFTER 6 WEEKS

Nellie Otero
Age 48 • Height 5 feet, 6.75 inches

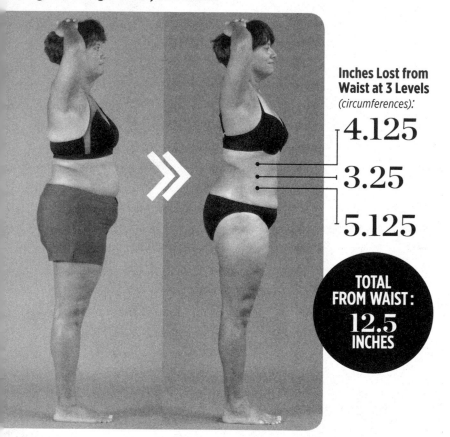

Inches Lost from Waist at 3 Levels
(circumferences):

4.125

3.25

5.125

TOTAL FROM WAIST: 12.5 INCHES

Weight Before: **196.7 pounds**
Weight After: **184.7 pounds**
FAT LOSS: 17.35 pounds
Muscle Gain: **5.35 pounds**

"My water bottle has become my best friend. It's the first thing I see in the morning and the last thing I see before bed."
—*Nellie Otero*

chapter
8
Just Add Walking

Sipping and Strolling Will Whittle Your Middle

Besides sipping ice water all day long, there's another routine I want you to practice on the Tighten Your Tummy program that will increase the daily calories you burn. Would you walk a mile for a meal? Well, that's exactly what I want you to do, except in reverse.

After your 300-calorie evening meal, I want you to walk about 1.5 miles at a leisurely pace. Let me explain.

Research shows that walking with food in your belly generates approximately 30 percent extra body heat. As you know, body heat means calories are being burned. Plus, if you carry your water bottle with you and sip 16 ounces of ice water during your stroll, you'll produce 40 or even 50 percent more body heat.

For example, the average 40-year-old woman who weighs 180 pounds can expect to burn approximately 218 calories in an evening applying this eating-walking-watering routine. Spread over 42 days, that would add up to 9,156 calories—or more than $2\frac{1}{2}$ pounds lost!

Remember, this is leisurely walking. I'm not asking you to run or even walk fast to get the benefit. The pace will help with digestion, and because it isn't strenuous, it will significantly reduce the load on the knee joints.

Here are the exact walking guidelines that all my test panel participants received at the start of the Tighten Your Tummy program. You should follow these as well.

- Eat your evening meal.

- Begin your walk within 15 minutes after you finish eating.

- Walk at a leisurely pace for 30 minutes. A leisurely pace should cover 1.5 miles, which translates to a speed of 3 miles an hour.

- Carry your insulated water bottle with you. Sip 16 ounces of ice water as you walk.

- Wear well-constructed, well-cushioned walking or running shoes. Do not wear street shoes.

- Dress in lightweight, comfortable clothes.

- Walk outdoors on level ground. Or you may substitute a bicycle ride for a walk. If the weather is a problem, you may walk indoors or use an exercise bike, treadmill, or elliptical.

- Do this each day for 42 consecutive days.

Apply my eating-walking-watering guidelines for the Tighten Your Tummy program and you'll be hooked on the after-dinner routine as a healthy habit for life.

My wife, Jeanenne, who is featured in the Introduction, has followed this routine almost every day for more than a year. She says walking and drinking a gallon of ice-cold water has helped her to lose 40 pounds of fat—and keep it off.

Many people who start the Tighten Your Tummy program feel some intimidation about drinking a gallon of water a day. That's understandable, because it is a bit out of the ordinary. Jeanenne felt that way, too. After all— water in necessitates water out, which can make long drives on highways more challenging. For this reason, I asked Jeanenne to share her experiences of drinking, walking . . . and running to the bathroom. Here's 24 hours in her life as a gallon-a-day drinker.

THE GALLON-A-DAY CLUB
A Day in the Life of a Heavy (ice water) Drinker

It was a year and a half ago that I adopted the regimen of drinking a gallon of ice-cold water daily. I've never been a big water drinker, ever. So when Ell laid out my program for fat loss, which included after-dinner walking and a gallon of water a day, I knew this was going to be a challenge. I was a coffee drinker for breakfast, sweet tea for lunch and dinner, and maybe a Diet Coke if I got thirsty in between. I never just drank water. Looking back, I'm sure I was walking around most of the time in a state of partial dehydration.

In retrospect, the only time in my life that I ever came close to drinking the proper amount of water was after the birth of our two children, Tyler, who is now 13, and Larah, who is 9. When I was nursing, I had to drink loads of water to ensure enough milk production, and I was dedicated to nursing my babies. Other than that, water was never my "go-to" drink. My hands and feet were always dry no matter how much lotion I used, and I tried them all! Ell had been telling me all along, "Jeanenne, you hydrate from the inside out!" I just never got it. I should have listened to him.

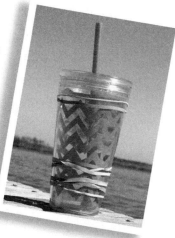

So at my heaviest point, 184.5 pounds and miserable, I had had enough and knew it was time to commit and get this fat off. Aside from moving to a 1,200-calorie-per-day eating plan, working out twice a week, walking 30 minutes after dinner, and getting extra sleep, I had to drink a gallon of water each day! So I picked up an insulated tumbler with a straw. I'd always heard it's easier to drink through a straw. The container actually holds 23 ounces of liquid, but when I load it with ice to the rim, it reduces the volume to 16 ounces. Some quick math of 16 into 128 told me I had to fill the glass eight times a day. WOW! I thought, "How am I ever going to get down that much water?"

I knew I had to find a way of keeping track of the exact amount I'd consumed, so I put eight rubber bands on the bottom of my tumbler to represent the eight times I had to refill my glass. Each time I finished 16 ounces, I moved one rubber band from the bottom up to the top of the glass. I wouldn't stop drinking until

Jeanenne's 23-ounce tumbler, with a straw and the necessary rubber bands. She's finished her second glass, moved the second rubber band to the top, and reloaded with ice and water. She's now ready for Round 3.

all the rubber bands were at the top of the glass. And the next morning, I would work in reverse and move them down to the bottom. So back and forth went my rubber bands to keep me honest. An added bonus I hadn't counted on, the rubber bands make the tumbler more secure in the car cup holder, and it doesn't rattle! We have to look for these little silver linings, right?

Needless to say, drinking all that water makes you pretty conscious of the location of restrooms wherever you go. Because you will go a lot. Here's what a regular day looks like for me, with a lot of bathroom breaks!

7:00 A.M. Alarm goes off. Boy, am I thirsty!

7:01 A.M. First trip to the bathroom.

7:05 A.M. Two cups of coffee to kick-start my day.

8:20 A.M. I fill my glass with ice, then top it off with water, and drive Larah to school. Sip, sip, sip!

9:20 A.M. Trot to my bathroom.

10:18 A.M. Reload on ice and water. Move one rubber band to the top of my tumbler. One glass down and seven to go. As I head to the mall, I guzzle most of the cold stuff on the way and finish as I park.

10:25 A.M. First stop, Macy's restroom.

11:00 A.M. Reload with ice and water at the food court. Sit for a bit and drink the whole glass. Move another rubber band to the rim.

11:10 A.M. Food court restroom.

11:15 A.M. Reload my water at Chick-Fil-A. More shopping. Slip another band up the rim.

11:30 A.M. Bloomingdale's pit stop. Love the marble bathrooms.

NOON Reload once again at Chick-Fil-A. They recognize me from my earlier trip. Time to slide another band up the cup. I'm right on schedule—it's a little after noon and I'm halfway to eight refills.

12:40 P.M. Slip into the Justice store bathroom while shopping for Larah. They recognize me there, too.

1:30 P.M. I fill up again at lunch. Scoot another band to the top. Now that I'm satisfied, it's safe to go to the grocery store.

1:45 P.M. First things first. Hit the restroom at Publix. It's always clean and familiar . . . very familiar . . .

2:15 P.M.   Meanwhile, back to the Publix restroom before I leave—and NOT by choice. Head home to meet Larah's bus.

2:50 P.M.   I'm done with public toilets for the day—I finally get to use my own bathroom this time!

3:05 P.M.   Another ice-cold refill, and I inch another band up the glass. I watch Larah get off the bus in front of our house, and we walk through our front door as I keep chugging.

4:04 P.M.   Bathroom break at home before heading back out.

4:10 P.M.   I reload with ice and water. Slide another band up the rim. Jump in the car and head off to Larah's piano lesson.

4:30 P.M.   Quick trip to the restroom at Larah's piano lesson.

5:15 P.M.   I'm halfway through the last 16 ounces, which means I'm at 120 ounces. I'll save the rest for my evening walk. I make dinner, and I'm not as hungry with all this water on board.

5:20 P.M.   Run to my own restroom again.

6:00 P.M.   Finish dinner and I head to the bathroom before slipping on my running shoes. I grab my bottle, fill it with a little more ice and water, and am off on my evening walk.

6:04 P.M.   Quick pit stop.

6:30 P.M.   Complete my walk and my water! I do the math: 128 plus 8 equals 136 ounces, so I'm a little over today, which is usual for me.

7:10 P.M.   Maybe it's doing the math, but I have to head to the bathroom again.

7:35 P.M.   Another trip to the restroom. Where is all this water coming from? I stopped drinking 2 hours ago!

8:30 P.M.   Got to go again!

9:30 P.M.   My post-bed pit stop.

1:35 A.M.   Middle-of-the-night awakening: my last bathroom break before morning. Phew!

At the end of the day, I tally 18 bathroom breaks total and surpass my water goal, logging 136 ounces!

BEFORE & AFTER 6 WEEKS

Marlene Hill

Age 59 • Height 5 feet, 6 inches

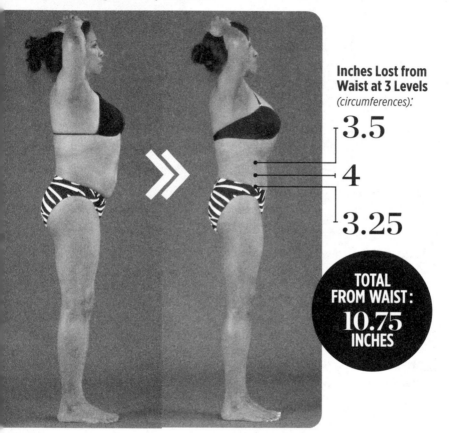

Inches Lost from Waist at 3 Levels
(circumferences):

3.5

4

3.25

TOTAL FROM WAIST:

10.75 INCHES

Weight Before: **157.7 pounds**

Weight After: **140.75 pounds**

FAT LOSS: 20.12 pounds

Muscle Gain: **3.17 pounds**

"I'm so happy that my belly has shrunk. Now, I feel much more alive and sexy."

—*Marlene Hill*

chapter

9

Master the Inner-Ab Vacuum

Your Most Valuable Tummy Tightener

Whenever I put a group of people through a fat-loss program, I typically invite them to a celebration at the end. It's a chance to review our results, celebrate the "biggest losers," and reflect back on the adventure while enjoying each other's company once more. After all, we've grown tight as a team.

The Tighten Your Tummy program was no different. Participants took center stage at a special event to celebrate the end of 6 weeks of hard work. And all of them came decked out in newly purchased clothes to fit their new bodies. They all looked amazing—like they were red carpet ready.

One extra-special guest and test panel participant that evening was my daughter, Sarah. At one point in the program, Sarah stood front and center among a sea of success stories and lifted her shirt to show off her pride in her perfectly toned tummy. The audience strained to see the smallness of a waist that measured exactly 24 inches!

Then Sarah demonstrated the move that all the participants knew well as a daily part of their Tighten Your Tummy to-do list: the "inner-ab vacuum." Sarah exhaled all the air from her lungs and then, by engaging her transverse abdominal muscle, pulled her stomach up and back. She straightened up, faced the audience, and hit them with a concave belly that looked as if it measured no more than 18 inches. "That's how you do an inner-ab vacuum," she said. Nobody does it quite like Sarah.

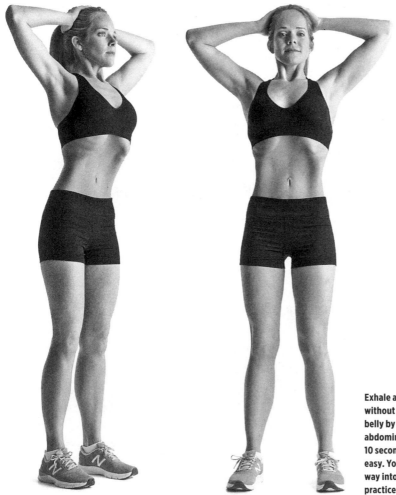

Exhale all the air you can. Then, without inhaling, pull in your belly by contracting your inner-abdominal muscle and hold for 10 seconds. Sarah makes it look easy. You may want to ease your way into the exercise with a few practice sessions.

The inner-ab vacuum, which you will learn how to do ahead, is performed twice before every meal on the Tighten Your Tummy program. Many of the test panelists found it extremely helpful, especially Sarah. She said the exercise improved her posture, eased her lower-back pain, and made her more aware of how filling her 300-calorie meals really felt. As a result, she lost more than 26 pounds and 15 inches off her waist. She credits the ab vacuum as her most important weapon in weight loss—and it only took her and her fellow participants a couple of practice sessions to master.

The Stomach Vacuum: An ABridged History

I learned the inner-ab vacuum (also referred to as the stomach vacuum) more than 50 years ago from a champion bodybuilder. In the 1960s, bodybuilding contests were not as popular as they are today. The state and regional contests were held mostly in small venues or in dusty basketball courts of YMCAs.

As a young, inexperienced bodybuilder, I remember the first time I saw the vacuum performed. It was 1964 at the YMCA in downtown Oklahoma City. I was the youngest contestant at just 20 years old, and Tuny Monday was the oldest, at 37. Tuny was 5 foot 5 and weighed 155 pounds, tanned and super ripped.

During Tuny's posing routine on the stage, he sucked in his stomach to such a degree that you could almost see his backbone from the front. Then he proceeded to pop out his cleanly defined abs one at a time from top to bottom. It was an impressive display of muscle control and was a key reason he won the competition.

After the contest, I asked him to teach me the move. It took me a while to get the techniques under control, but over the next several shows, I was able to pull off the stomach vacuum and master ab muscle control. Eventually, it helped me win several bodybuilding competitions.

Inner-Ab Anatomy

Have you ever noticed those thick, heavy belts that some competitive weight lifters (and even workers at Home Depot) wear prior to lifting something heavy? Those belts aren't a macho fashion accessory. Cinched tightly, they add support to the spine and midsection, which is useful for avoiding injury when lifting a heavy object.

Similarly, your inner-ab muscles, also known as your transverse abdominals, act as a natural weight belt. When it contracts, it increases inner-abdominal pressure to support your spine.

These muscles aren't just good for when you have to lift something heavy like a barbell; they are also responsible for keeping your organs in place. Strengthening them isn't just for vanity purposes.

Vacuuming 101: Master the "Suck"

You may have shimmied your way into skinny jeans or "sucked it in" to inch your zipper to the top of your favorite dress, but now it's time to take the common phrase and put it to proper practice. To master the vacuum, start with these steps:

- Have an empty belly.

- Lie in bed on your back.

- Place your hands on the bottom of your rib cage, at the top of your abdominals.

- Take a normal breath and forcibly blow out as much air as possible for about 7 to 8 seconds.

- Next, suck in your stomach to the maximum degree using your inner-abdominal muscles. You should feel as if you are trying to suck your navel into your backbone. Do not breathe in air during this process; use only your ab muscles.

- You should feel a concave formation under your rib cage. This concave feel and look is the effect of the stomach vacuum. You will not be able to hold this position very long, probably no longer than 10 seconds.

- Try the vacuum several more times while lying down. If you experience a little light-headedness, that's normal. Rest a bit longer between attempts.

- Now stand and move in front of a mirror to try the vacuum. Because of the forces of gravity, the vacuum is more difficult to do in a standing position. But with a little practice, you'll be able to master it.

- Work on learning the inner-ab vacuum for 3 consecutive days for about 15 minutes each day.

After about 3 days of practice, you should be able to perform the stomach vacuum standing up. Practice it twice before breakfast, lunch, and dinner—or six times a day—for the first 2 weeks. Continue to do the inner-ab vacuum six times a day for the duration of the Tighten Your Tummy program, and the involved muscles will become even stronger and more under your control.

BEFORE & AFTER 6 WEEKS

Brianna Kramer
Age 23 • Height 5 feet, 6.5 inches

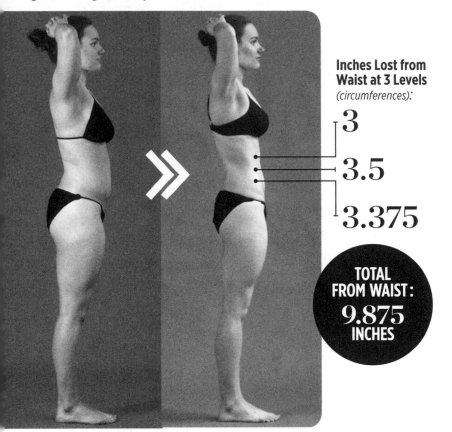

Inches Lost from Waist at 3 Levels
(circumferences):

3

3.5

3.375

TOTAL FROM WAIST: 9.875 INCHES

Weight Before: **152.1 pounds**
Weight After: **134.1 pounds**
FAT LOSS: 20.86 pounds
Muscle Gain: **2.86 pounds**

"I wasted so much time attempting to get my body in shape by doing more and more exercise. The twice-a-week, negative-accentuated training proved to me that less is better."

—Brianna Kramer

chapter
10
Exercises for a Flat Belly

Lose Fat with a Special Training Plan

I know you are anxious to start exercising. And you won't be disappointed. This chapter explains the Tighten Your Tummy strength-building workouts that are designed to accelerate the loss of belly fat. You will like them because they are simple and effective, you can do them in your home, and they don't take up a lot of your precious time.

The exercise program requires only two strength workouts per week. Each will take you about 20 minutes. The exercises are simple moves that require either a pair of lightweight dumbbells or no equipment at all. They are the same exercises that my test panels in Gainesville used. There is one special piece of equipment that I highly recommend but is not essential to the Tighten Your Tummy program. I've included it because my test panels used it very effectively, and I believe that you will see better and faster results if you use it. It's available for purchase nationwide for under $39. You'll learn more about it later in this chapter. But again, I want to stress that it is not required.

Before you begin, there are a few important points about strength training that you need to understand.

You Can Reduce Your Trouble Spots

Many people believe that when you exercise a specific body part, such as the abdominals or legs, the involved muscles burn the surrounding fat for energy. This is commonly known as spot reduction. Research shows, however, that there are no direct pathways from the muscle cells to the fat cells. When fat is used for energy, it is mobilized primarily through the liver from fat cells located all over the body. So, the thinking goes, doing situps won't burn belly fat. That belief is accepted by scientists all over the world, and I've supported that thinking for years.

But in 2012, while during research for *The Body Fat Breakthrough,* I observed something that seemed very close to spot reduction in many of the men and women in my exercise study. I found that nearly all of them lost a disproportionate amount of belly fat, as opposed to overall body fat. I also experienced the phenomenon in my own body from the same special type of strength training that my test panelists were doing. It wasn't necessarily situp exercises that were spot-reducing belly fat, but something else was happening to eliminate more fat from the abdominal region.

Naturally curious, I reviewed the most current exercise research to see if there were any clues to explain what might be occurring. There were, in fact, several.

Researchers in the early 2000s began exploring the unique secretions deep inside working muscles, especially when muscles were subjected to heavy negative exercise. Remember, "negative" or eccentric exercise emphasizes the lowering portion of a resistance exercise, and it is typically done slower than the positive phase of an exercise. The natural chemicals produced by these muscles under stress are called myokines, and they are important because they act like hormones, causing reactions in the body. The researchers eventually further classified these secretions as interleukins—namely, interleukin-6, interleukin-8, and interleukin-15. Interleukin-15 is of particular importance because it causes muscle-fat cross talk. Put simply, under the right conditions, it promotes muscle building and the loss of fat.

What I witnessed in those test subjects suggests to me that it may be possible to spot-reduce your body fat under these specific circumstances: (1) if you use the negative-accentuated technique to exercise the muscles underlying the fat you want to get rid of; and (2) if you eat a lower-calorie, carbohydrate-rich diet during your training.

In 2014, I retested these two conditions with 41 women for the book you are holding in your hands. As expected, these test subjects also lost a large amount of fat from their midsections.

Naturally, much more research needs to be done, but for now I'm excited about what I've observed in the test subjects in Gainesville. I believe you will also lose pounds and inches from your tummy by teaming a low-calorie diet with the negative-accentuated exercises in this chapter.

Muscle Isolation

The negative-accentuated routines you'll learn here isolate your abdominals and work those muscles intensely. But that doesn't mean they neglect other major muscles in your body. On the contrary, you'll be exercising your entire body, especially the other important muscle groups of your hips, thighs, shoulders, chest, and arms.

If you combine one of the routines in this chapter with the diet plan, the superhydration guidelines, the rest/sleep schedule, and the other steps in this program, then you've done everything practical—just short of liposuction—to achieve a flat tummy.

Important Guidelines
for the Exercise Routines

Read through them first: Spend several minutes examining the exercises in this chapter. Read the instructions carefully. Practice will perfect your movements, but for now do them as best you can.

Exercise at home: There's no need to join a fitness club or gym if you don't wish to. The negative-accentuated routine in this chapter is designed to be performed in the privacy of your own home using only your own body weight and, for two exercises, a pair of lightweight dumbbells. If you already have a roller-type abdominal machine, such as the Ab Roller Evolution shown in this book, or you wish to purchase one, I've included instructions and photos to help you incorporate it into your workout routine. The Ab Roller is useful for doing some negative-accentuated exercises. But you'll soon find that the equipment is not nearly as important as the way in which you perform an exercise. Remember this: Slow, controlled movement is critical for success.

Apply negative-accentuated repetitions: As I've mentioned, the negative or lowering portion of each repetition is the most important and should be emphasized when possible. Let's explore how to do it using the 15-15-15 technique that I introduced in Chapter 5. You will begin an exercise in the contracted or "up" position and do a 15-second negative, followed by a 15-second positive, and another 15-second negative. You can try counting the seconds, but it's a lot easier and more accurate to use a wristwatch with a stopwatch function or have a clock in the room. Even better yet: Ask a partner to time you.

Let's follow a simple pushup through these steps: You start in the up position, with arms straight, and gradually lower yourself toward the floor, taking 15 seconds to do so, then push back up to the starting position for 15 seconds, and again lower yourself for 15 seconds. You're finished with the negative-accentuated part of the exercise. Now, you immediately do 8 repetitions at normal exercise speed—1 second up and 2 seconds down equals one repetition. Stop and rest after the last pushup.

Remember to breathe as you do these exercises. Don't hold your breath! When the movement becomes difficult, purse your lips and exhale in short bursts, just like they teach in a Lamaze class.

Rest between workouts and progress: This is important: Always rest for at least 2 days before doing the second workout of the week. Your recovery time is essential for muscle growth and fat loss. Then, on each successive workout, increase the regular-speed repetitions by one. That's what we call progression, and it's another way you build strength. Thus, if you begin your first workout on Monday, the progression would be as follows:

WEEK 1

> **Monday:** 15-15-15, 8 repetitions for all exercises
>
> **Thursday:** 15-15-15, 9 repetitions for all exercises

WEEK 2

> **Monday:** 15-15-15, 10 repetitions for all exercises
>
> **Thursday:** 15-15-15, 11 repetitions for all exercises

WEEK 3

> **Monday:** 15-15-15, 12 repetitions for all exercises
>
> **Thursday:** Add 5 percent to resistance; 15-15-15, 8 repetitions for all exercises

After you can do 12 or more perfect repetitions, you must add 5 percent more resistance to your body. This in turn will reduce your repetitions down to 8 or 9 at the next workout. Then it's your job to progress up to 12 repetitions once again and add another 5 percent, and so on.

Focus your concentration: Negative-accentuated strength training is both physical and mental. If you direct your attention to the muscles you are targeting, your results will improve. If doing a forward crunch, for example, focus on your front abdominals. Try to visualize them lengthening and shortening each time you lower your shoulders slowly to the floor and lift your shoulders smoothly to the top position. If doing an obliques crunch, focus on mobilizing your oblique muscles on your sides to their maximum. Aim your mind like a laser beam. The effect will amaze you.

Anticipate some soreness: Soreness in your body is an indicator that you've stretched and contracted underutilized muscles. Expect some tenderness after your first workout, especially on the front and sides of your waist. Don't fret. Your second workout will ease the soreness, and it should be gone by your third session.

Warm up and cool down: Before your negative-accentuated workout, take several minutes to warm up. A good way to do this is to walk in place. Start lifting your feet and hands in a slow, walking-in-place motion. After 1 minute, gradually increase the range by lifting your hands to the level of your ears. Practice this exaggerated action for another minute. After your workout, cool down by walking around the exercise area, getting a drink of water, and moving your arms in slow circles. Continue these easy actions for several minutes until your heart rate slows down.

Those are the pointers. Now you can start practicing the exercises. Here is the progressive 6-week schedule of two workouts a week. You can expect to feel and see the greatest results in the first 2 weeks on the Tighten Your Tummy program.

The Workouts

For the first 2 weeks of the program, no special equipment is needed. During Weeks 3 through 6, you will add exercises requiring the use of a pair of lightweight dumbbells.

Weeks 1 and 2: Perform 1 set (that's $1\frac{1}{2}$ slow reps at 15-15-15 seconds plus 8 regular-speed repetitions) of the following:

Forward Crunch

Obliques Crunch (left and right)

V-Crunch

Pushup

Squat

Weeks 3 and 4: Add 1 set of the following to your routine: Dumbbell Curl (15-15-15 plus 8 regular-speed reps)

Weeks 5 and 6: Add one set of the following to your routine: Dumbbell Overhead Press (15-15-15 plus 8 regular-speed reps)

Body Weight and Dumbbell Exercises

All you'll need for the following exercises are a watch with a second hand, a pair of dumbbells, and an exercise mat.

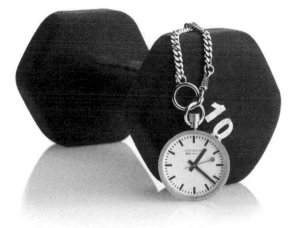

Forward Crunch

MUSCLES WORKED: RECTUS ABDOMINIS

Preparation

Lie on your back with your knees bent about 90 degrees, feet flat on the floor and close together (your knees should be touching).

Clasp your fingers and extend your arms in front of your navel.

Keep your feet firmly planted as you lift your shoulders off the ground, contracting your abdominal muscles. This is the starting position.

First Negative

Contract your abdominals intensely and hold tight. Viewed from the side, your torso should be approximately 45 degrees off the floor.

Start lowering your shoulders slowly. You should be about halfway to the floor at 10 seconds. Focus. Relax your face and neck, and don't hold your breath. Lower another inch until your shoulders barely touch the floor at 15 seconds.

Prepare to lift your shoulders off the ground again to the starting position.

Positive

Start to crunch upward slowly, ½ inch by ½ inch. You should be halfway to your starting position after 10 seconds and all the way to the top at 15 seconds. Pause briefly at the top, in the contracted position.

Second Negative

Slowly lower your shoulders to the floor. Aim to be halfway to the floor after 10 seconds. Your shoulders should reach the bottom at 15 seconds.

Regular Reps

Do 8 to 12 normal-speed repetitions, taking 1 second for the positive and 2 seconds for the negative.

When you can do 12 repetitions easily, try switching your hand position to make the exercise harder. See the descriptions of the hand position variations on page 86.

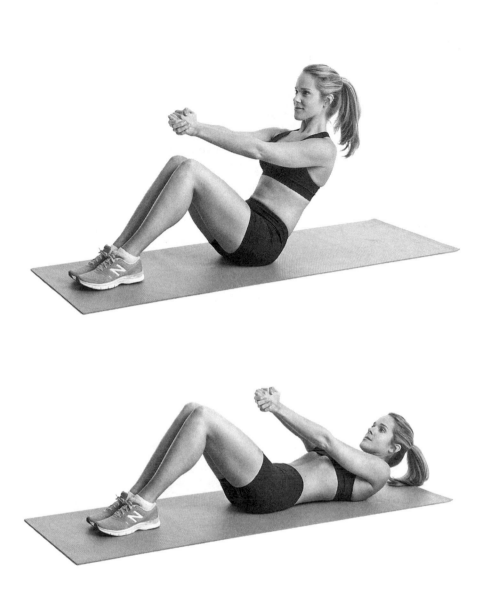

TIPS
- *Stabilize your torso and arms as you move your shoulders and torso down and up.*
- *Do not pull with your hands and arms. Focus on crunching your abdominals.*

Forward Crunch Variations

The slow negative-accentuated half repetitions (two negatives and a positive) make a deeper inroad into your starting level of strength, which triggers at least six tummy-tightening hormones that affect fat burn. The 8 to 12 faster repetitions, done after you've already taxed your muscles, reinforce that pulsating biochemistry. Progressing your exercises—that is, making them more difficult—is one way to continue to trigger those fat-burning hormones.

Where you place your hands and arms during the forward crunch will make the exercise easier or harder.

Beginner Hand Position

Everyone should master the basic forward crunch before changing hand positions. You learned this on the previous page, but here it is again. The basic learning position is with your arms extended over your navel and your hands clasped. This places some of the weight of your hands and arms forward, which decreases the resistance against your torso, making the crunch easier to do.

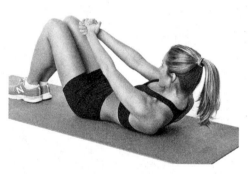

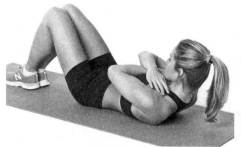

Crossed-Hand Position

The first progression for a harder forward crunch is to cross your hands over your chest. Have your fingertips touch your shoulders. This moves some of the weight of your hands and arms from your navel to your chest, adding more resistance to your torso.

Over-Ear Position

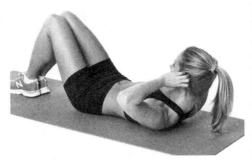

This tougher progression will shift the weight of your hands and arms from your chest to your head area. Do not interlace your hands behind your head or neck. Doing so can strain your neck by pulling forward on your head. Instead, cup your hands around your ears while keeping your elbows back and at shoulder level. Your hands and arms in this position make the forward crunch significantly harder than the first two versions.

Weighted Crunch

The most difficult progression adds weight to your torso. Hold a 2½- or 5-pound weight plate or lightweight dumbbell (as shown) over your upper chest. This will add significant resistance to your crunch. If your abs become so strong that even this is easy, simply increase the weight to make it harder.

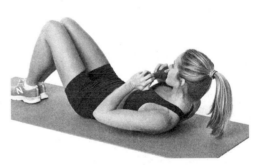

Adjust the toughness!

EASIER: MOVE FASTER THAN 15-15-15. TRY 10-10-10. Afterward, do fewer than 8 repetitions.

HARDER: MOVE SLOWER THAN 15-15-15. TRY 20-20-20. Change the position of your arms and hands. Hold a small weight plate (5 pounds) across your chest.

Obliques Crunch

MUSCLES WORKED: OBLIQUES AND RECTUS ABDOMINIS

Preparation

Lie on your back with your knees bent about 90 degrees, feet flat. Drop your knees to the floor on your left side, stacking your right leg on top of your left. Keep your shoulders flat on the ground. Clasp your fingers and extend your arms toward your right hip. Lift your shoulders off the floor quickly, twisting smoothly to the left and trying to touch your hands to your right knee. Pause.

First Negative

Contract your abdominals and right-side obliques intensely as you start to slowly lower your shoulders. You should be approximately halfway to the floor at the 10-second mark. At 15 seconds, your shoulders should be untwisted and flat, hovering just about an inch above the floor.

Positive

Return to the top ever so slowly, $\frac{1}{2}$ inch by $\frac{1}{2}$ inch. You should be twisting left and halfway up at 10 seconds and all the way to the top at 15 seconds.

Pause briefly in the contracted position at the top before starting the second negative.

Second Negative

Take 15 seconds to slowly lower your shoulders to the floor, contracting your abdominals and right-side obliques, as before.

Regular Reps

Do 8 to 12 normal-speed repetitions. Do them smoothly with good form, taking 1 second for the positive and 2 seconds for the negative.

Don't compromise your form. Start with a goal of 8 perfect crunches until you feel you can add more. Relax after the last repetition and then repeat the exercise with your legs on the floor to your right side.

 • *Focus on uncrunching and crunching your abdominals.*

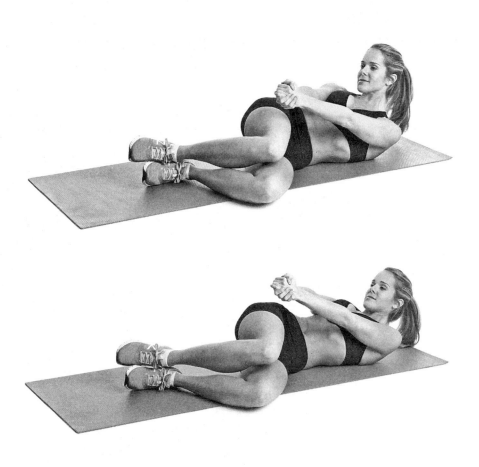

Adjust the toughness!

EASIER: DO EACH SLOW PHASE FOR 10 seconds instead of 15, then do fewer regular reps.

HARDER: TAKE 20 SECONDS FOR EACH slow phase or hold a small weight plate across your chest.

V-Crunch

MUSCLES WORKED: RECTUS ABDOMINIS
(you'll feel it more in the lower area)

Preparation

Lie on your back with your knees bent about 90 degrees, feet flat on the floor and close together (your knees should be touching). Clasp your fingers and extend your arms in front of your navel.

Raise your legs straight in the air, in line with your hips and perpendicular to your torso. The soles of your feet should point toward the ceiling. Keep your feet and legs in that position for the duration of the exercise. Have a watch or big clock with a second hand in plain sight to keep track of timing on your slow reps.

Raise your shoulders and torso off the ground, contracting your abs intensely. This is the starting position.

First Negative

In the top crunch position, contract your abdominals intensely, then start lowering your shoulders slowly.

You should be approximately halfway down at 10 seconds. Lower another few inches slowly until you barely touch the floor at 15 seconds.

Positive

Start the positive V-crunch slowly, ½ inch by ½ inch. You should be halfway up at 10 seconds and all the way to the top at 15 seconds.

Keep your legs and feet pointing straight up. Do not let them sag. Pause briefly in the contracted position.

Second Negative

Repeat the procedure for the first negative. Try to be halfway down at 10 seconds and at the bottom at 15 seconds.

Regular Reps

Do 8 to 12 normal-speed repetitions, taking 1 second for the positive and 2 seconds for the negative.

- *Stabilize your torso and arms as you move down and up.*
- *Do not push with your hands and arms. Concentrate the movement on your abdominals.*

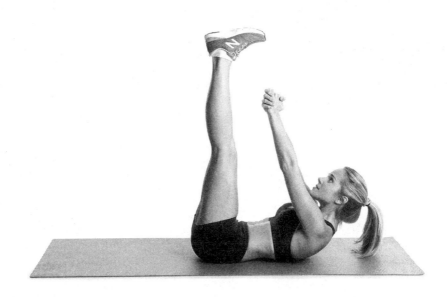

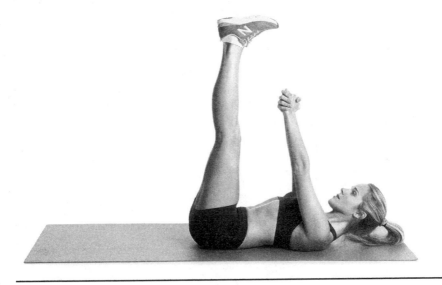

Adjust the toughness!

EASIER: MOVE FASTER THAN 15-15-15. TRY 10-10-10. Or do fewer than 8 normal-speed repetitions.

HARDER: MOVE SLOWER THAN 15-15-15. TRY 20-20-20. Change the position of your arms and hands as in the forward crunch variations (see page 86). Hold a small weight plate (5 pounds) across your chest.

Pushup

MUSCLES WORKED: PECTORALIS MAJOR, DELTOIDS, AND TRICEPS

Preparation

Assume a pushup position on your toes, positioning your feet close together, with your body off the floor and your arms fully extended. Place your hands shoulder-width apart, with your thumbs to the inside.

Keep your legs, hips, midsection, and lower back rigid. There should be a straight line from your ankles to your head, with a slight S curve in your lower back.

Your goal is to lower, raise, and lower your body as a unit very slowly, approximately 2 inches with each 5-second count. Have a watch with a second hand in plain sight so you can pace yourself, or get a spotter to stand nearby to help with the counting.

First Negative

Hold the top position briefly before you start. Then bend your elbows slightly and lower your body just a little. Continue to bend and lower inch by inch. You should be approximately halfway down at 10 seconds.

Focus. Relax your face and neck and don't hold your breath. In fact, breathe often. You should be at the bottom at 15 seconds.

Keep your chin and hips up. Your chest should barely graze the floor as you smoothly begin the positive phase.

Positive

Start the positive pushing slowly, 1 inch by 1 inch. Keep your focus and continue breathing. You should be halfway up at 10 seconds.

Continue pushing with your arms and chest muscles. Don't let your elbows flare out. Keep them near your torso. You should be at the top at 15 seconds.

Second Negative

Repeat the procedure for the first negative. Bend your elbows slightly and lower inch by inch. Try to be halfway down at 10 seconds. Touch your chest to the floor at 15 seconds.

Regular Reps

Immediately start doing regular reps. Perform these smoothly, taking 1 second for the positive and 2 seconds for the negative.

Push yourself to complete 8 repetitions. Relax after the last repetition.

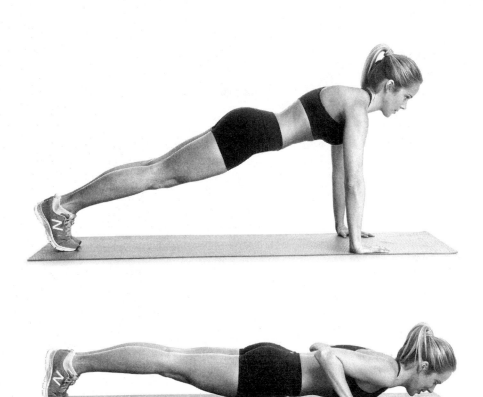

 • *Be aware of your body (or have a friend watch you) to make sure you maintain a straight, rigid back throughout the exercise.*

Adjust the toughness!

EASIER: REDUCE THE TIME UNDER TENSION to 10 seconds for the negative-accentuated phase. Do fewer than 8 regular reps. Or do the pushup with your hands on a bench that's at hip height, which will make your body form a 45-degree angle to the floor, significantly reducing the resistance.

HARDER: INCREASE THE TIME UNDER LOAD to 20 seconds. Or wear a weighted vest.

Squat

MUSCLES WORKED: HAMSTRINGS, QUADRICEPS, AND GLUTEALS

Preparation

Stand straight and place your feet a little wider than shoulder-width apart, with your toes angled out slightly. Clasp your hands in front of your chest, with your elbows up and out. Doing so will help you keep your balance as you bend your knees. As you get stronger, you may want to hold a dumbbell between your hands goblet-style. Have a watch with a second hand in plain sight so you can pace yourself to keep track of time on your slow reps.

First Negative

Start bending your knees slightly, first 1 inch, then 2 inches.

Slowly and smoothly push your hips and butt back as if you were going to close a door behind you with your butt. Keep a slight arch in your lower back.

You should be halfway down at 10 seconds. Breathe as you squat lower, with your fingers touching the wall if needed for balance. Go as low as you can without lifting your heels. Be at your lowest squat at 15 seconds.

Positive

Push down through your heels, not your toes, as you inch your way up. You should feel an intense contraction in your thighs.

Keep your head and shoulders up and focus on your breathing. You should be nearing the halfway-up position at 10 seconds.

Continue the slow, inch-by-inch ascent. Your hands are helping you balance.

Stand erect at the 15-second mark.

Second Negative

Repeat the slow lowering, inch by inch. Focus, breathe, and keep your core rigid. You should be halfway down at 10 seconds. The hardest part is from halfway down to the bottom.

Exert through your heels and fight gravity. At 15 seconds, simply stand erect.

Regular Reps

Immediately begin the 8 to 12 faster repetitions. Perform these smoothly, taking 1 second for the positive and 2 seconds for the negative phases of each rep. Push yourself to do 8 repetitions. Relax after the last repetition.

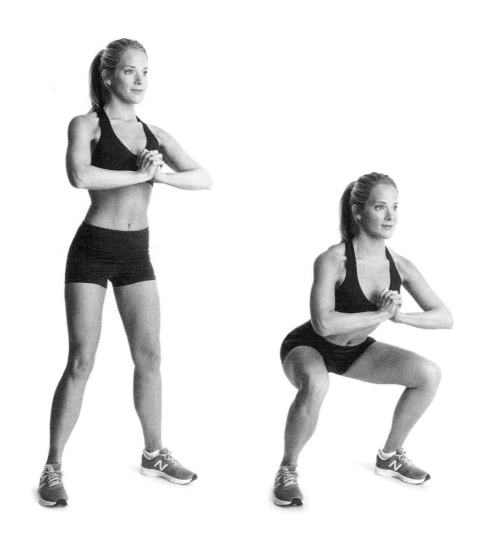

TIPS • *Note that your shape and flexibility can affect how deeply you squat.*

• *Some people have difficulty squatting below a level where the tops of their thighs are parallel to the floor. Others can almost touch their buttocks to their heels. If your ankles are tight and you tend to lift your heels at the bottom of the squat, try placing a 1-inch board under your heels for stability.*

Dumbbell Curl

MUSCLES WORKED: BICEPS

Preparation

Grasp a dumbbell in each hand and stand with your feet about shoulder-width apart. Most women feel comfortable starting with 5- or 10-pound dumbbells. As you stand, use some upward momentum and curl the weight to your shoulders. Anchor your elbows firmly against your sides. Keep a watch or big clock within eyesight to keep track of your timing on slow reps.

First Negative

Lower the dumbbells slowly, 1 inch by 1 inch. Reach the halfway-down position at 10 seconds.

Keep your torso erect as you reach the bottom position at 15 seconds.

Positive

From the bottom position, immediately begin curling the dumbbells up. Stabilize your elbows as you slowly lift the dumbbells to the halfway point at the 10-second mark.

Keep moving $\frac{1}{2}$ inch by $\frac{1}{2}$ inch. Pause in the top position at 15 seconds, but do not move your elbows forward. Keep them anchored against the sides of your waist.

Second Negative

Start the final descent and progress $\frac{1}{2}$ inch by $\frac{1}{2}$ inch. Be halfway down at 10 seconds.

Keep your elbows anchored firmly against your sides. Reach the bottom at 15 seconds.

Regular Reps

Perform 8 dumbbell curls smoothly at normal speed, taking 1 second for the positive and 2 seconds for the negative.

Push yourself and complete 8 repetitions. Place the dumbbells on the floor and relax.

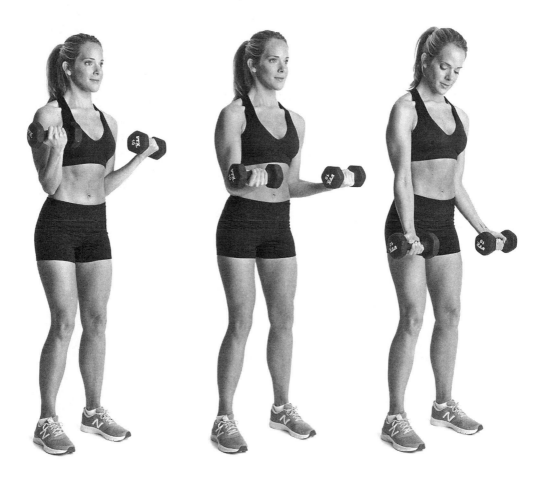

TIP • *Maximize your biceps stimulation by minimizing your body sway. Do not lean forward excessively or lean backward. Do not move your upper arms. Move only your hands, your forearms, and the dumbbells.*

Dumbbell Overhead Press

MUSCLES WORKED: DELTOIDS AND TRICEPS

Preparation

Choose a pair of light dumbbells. Five- to 10-pound dumbbells are ideal.

Place your feet shoulder-width apart, bend your knees slightly, and quickly press the dumbbells overhead. The dumbbells should be shoulder-width apart, and unlike a barbell that runs lengthwise across your shoulders, the dumbbells should be held parallel to each other, your palms facing each other. This is known as a neutral grip. Keep a watch or big clock within eyesight to keep track of your timing on slow reps.

First Negative

Lower the dumbbells slowly, inch by inch. Reach the halfway-down position at 10 seconds.

Keep the dumbbells apart and parallel to each other. Touch the dumbbells to your shoulders at 15 seconds.

Positive

Now press the dumbbells up slowly and smoothly, inch by inch. Be halfway up at 10 seconds.

Lock your elbows at 15 seconds. The dumbbells should still be parallel to each other.

Second Negative

Repeat the procedure for the first negative. Guide the dumbbells down slowly, inch by inch.

Move past the halfway point at 10 seconds. Touch the dumbbells to your shoulders at 15 seconds.

Regular Reps

Begin your regular-speed dumbbell presses smoothly, taking 1 second for the positive and 2 seconds for the negative. Try to complete 8 repetitions.

Place the dumbbells on the floor and relax.

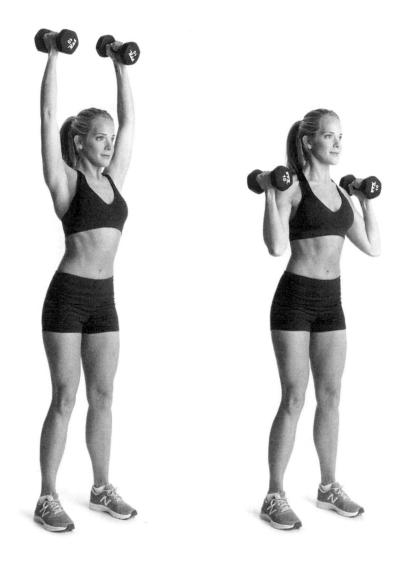

 TIPS
- *Keep your lower back naturally arched during the movements.*
- *It may take you several sessions to learn the mechanics of the negative-accentuated dumbbell overhead press, but it will be well worth it.*

Bonus Workout

Exercises with Ab Roller

The following workout is not required for the Tighten Your Tummy program, but my test panelists used it very effectively. I include it here in case you own an Ab Roller device or wish to purchase one online or at retail stores like Walmart. I did early research on the Ab Roller Evolution and found it helped people execute crunches with better form, which translated into better results.

The Ab Roller Evolution was invented by a man named Don Brown. I met Don in the early '90s, when he owned a large fitness center in Chester, New Jersey. He was a brilliant inventor who was looking for new ways to incorporate fitness in his ideas. He showed me a new machine designed for home use called the Ab Trainer. I tested it and liked the way it felt, so I told Don to send a few to Gainesville Health & Fitness and I'd test them out in my next fitness project. It's hard to believe that was 25 years ago! When it comes to exercise equipment, he's one of the most creative guys I've ever met. I've tested and trained people with his Ab Trainer, Ab Coaster, and most recently, the Ab Roller Evolution.

In June 2014, when I was telling Don about the Tighten Your Tummy test program, he suggested the Ab Roller Evolution because of its versatility. On one side, it's an on-the-floor abdominal machine that supports your head and neck for intense midsection exercise. Turn the machine over, and you can do pushups, dips, and even squats.

Don tested it with people of various fitness levels, but he was excited to see how the negative training would affect results. So 40 Ab Roller Evolution machines came to my doorstep in August 2014, and I organized two groups of women from Gainesville Health & Fitness to progress through a 6-week program using the Ab Roller. With the help of Joe Cirulli, Ann Raulerson, Lydia Maree, Jim Lennon, and personal trainer Pam Harrison, the program progressed in an orderly fashion.

Don and his crew from Tara Productions came to Gainesville to video the before-and-after measurements and interview the test panel of women involved in our research.

Again, the body weight and dumbbell workout described on the previous pages is the only workout you need to achieve great results. However, if you have an Ab Roller, you can use this workout instead. Or do one of your two weekly workouts with the Ab Roller and one without.

Ab Roller Exercises

For Weeks 1 and 2: Perform 1 set of five exercises, twice a week. Leave 2 days of rest between workouts.

Ab Roller Forward Crunch

Ab Roller Obliques Crunch (left and right)

Ab Roller V-Crunch

Ab Roller Pushup

Ab Roller Squat

For Weeks 3 and 4: Add the following exercise:

Dumbbell Curl

For Weeks 5 and 6: Add the following exercise:

Dumbbell Overhead Press

Ab Roller Forward Crunch

MUSCLES WORKED: RECTUS ABDOMINIS

Preparation

Set up the Ab Roller Evolution on a flat, level surface. The head and neck pad should be resting on the floor away from you. Keep a watch or big clock in sight, to keep track of your time on slow reps. Lie on your back and slide into the Ab Roller. Rest the back of your head and neck on the foam support. Bend your knees to 90 degrees and securely plant your feet on the floor. Place your hands on the top bar above your head. Crunch yourself into the up position. Your torso should be at about a 45-degree angle from the floor.

First Negative

From the top crunch position, contract your abdominals intensely and hold tight. Start lowering your shoulders slowly. You should be about halfway down at 10 seconds.

Focus. Relax your face and neck, and don't hold your breath. In fact, breathe often. Lower another inch until your shoulders barely touch the floor at 15 seconds.

Positive

Start the positive crunch slowly, $\frac{1}{2}$ inch by $\frac{1}{2}$ inch. You should be halfway up at 10 seconds and all the way to the top at 15 seconds.

Second Negative

Repeat the procedure for the first negative. Try to be halfway down at 10 seconds and at the bottom at 15 seconds.

Regular Reps

Progress immediately into 8 to 12 normal repetitions. Perform them at regular speed, taking 1 second for the positive and 2 seconds for the negative.

- *Stabilize your torso and arms as you move the Ab Roller forward and backward.*
- *Do not push with your hands and arms. Focus on crunching your abdominals and moving from the core.*

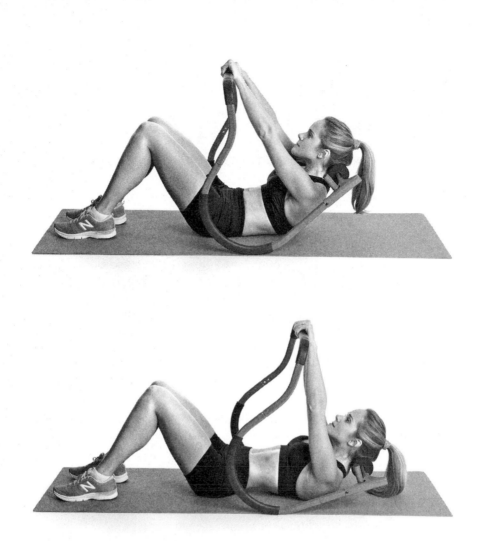

Adjust the toughness!

EASIER: DO THE NEGATIVE-ACCENTUATED PHASE faster, say 10 seconds, 10 seconds, 10 seconds. Afterward, do fewer regular-speed repetitions.

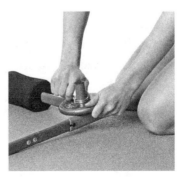

HARDER: ADD SMALL WEIGHT PLATES to the vertical posts on either side of the Ab Roller device.

Ab Roller Obliques Crunch

MUSCLES WORKED: OBLIQUES AND RECTUS ABDOMINIS

Preparation

Set up the Ab Roller Evolution on a flat, level surface. The head and neck pad should be resting on the floor away from you. Lie on your back and slide into the Ab Roller. Rest the back of your head and neck on the foam support. Bend your knees to 90 degrees and securely plant your feet on the floor.

Stack your knees and legs on the left side, which will stretch the right oblique muscles. Keep your shoulders flat on the ground. Place your right hand on the middle of the top bar above and your left hand in the top left side of the bar, close to the corner. Have a watch or big clock within eyesight to help keep track of timing your slower reps. Move to the top position quickly and pause.

First Negative

Intensely contract your abdominals and right-side obliques. Start lowering your shoulders slowly. You should be approximately halfway down at 10 seconds. Lower another inch until you barely touch the floor at 15 seconds.

Positive

Start the positive obliques crunch slowly, ½ inch by ½ inch. You should be halfway up at 10 seconds and all the way to the top at 15 seconds.

Pause briefly in the contracted up position.

Second Negative

Repeat the procedure for the first negative. Try to be halfway down at 10 seconds and at the bottom at 15 seconds.

Regular Reps

Progress immediately into 8 to 12 normal repetitions. Perform them smoothly at regular speed, taking approximately 1 to 2 seconds for the positive and 2 seconds for the negative. Rest a few seconds, then repeat the exercise on the other side with your legs stacked and lowered to the floor on the right side.

TIPS

- *Stabilize your torso and arms as you move the Ab Roller forward and backward. Do not push with your hands and arms. Focus on crunching your abdominals.*

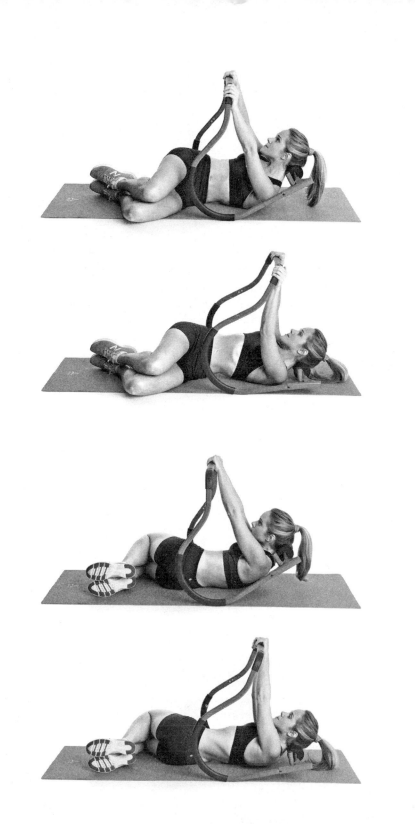

Ab Roller V-Crunch

MUSCLES WORKED: RECTUS ABDOMINIS

(you'll feel it more in the lower area)

Preparation

Set up the Ab Roller Evolution on a flat, level surface. The head and neck pad should be resting on the floor away from you. Lie on your back and slide into the Ab Roller. Rest the back of your head and neck on the foam support. Bend your knees to 90 degrees and securely plant your feet on the floor.

Raise your feet and legs so they are above your hips and perpendicular to your torso. The soles of your feet should face toward the ceiling. Keep your feet and legs in that position for the duration of the exercise. Have a watch or big clock within eyesight to help keep track of timing your slower reps. Raise your shoulders and torso to the top position quickly and pause.

First Negative

Contract your abdominals intensely. Start lowering your shoulders slowly. You should be approximately halfway down at 10 seconds.

Lower another inch until you barely touch the floor at 15 seconds.

Positive

Start the positive V-crunch slowly, ½ inch by ½ inch. You should be halfway up at 10 seconds and all the way to the top at 15 seconds.

Keep your legs and feet pointing straight up. Do not let them sag. Pause briefly in the contracted position.

Second Negative

Repeat the procedure for the first negative. Try to be halfway down at 10 seconds and at the bottom at 15 seconds.

Regular Reps

Perform 8 to 12 regular-speed repetitions smoothly, taking approximately 1 to 2 seconds for the positive and 2 seconds for the negative.

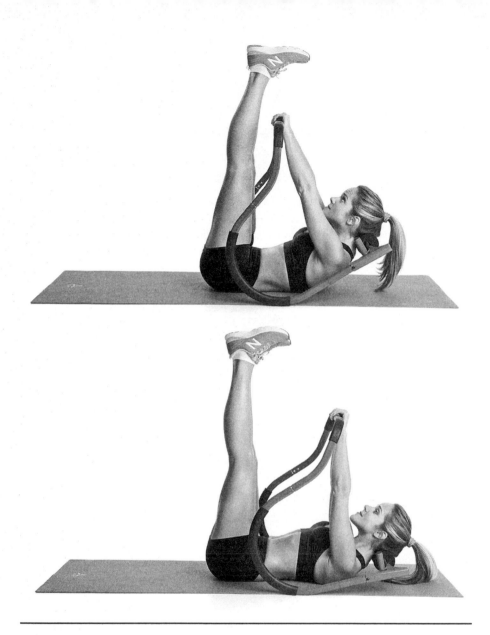

Adjust the toughness!

EASIER: MOVE FASTER THAN 15-15-15. TRY 10-10-10. Afterward, do fewer than 8 repetitions.

HARDER: MOVE SLOWER THAN 15-15-15. TRY 20-20-20. Add small plates (2.5 or 5 pounds) on the weight posts on the back of the Ab Roller.

Ab Roller Pushup

MUSCLES WORKED: PECTORALIS MAJOR, DELTOIDS, AND TRICEPS

Preparation

Using the Ab Roller for pushups is similar to placing your hands on a bench. It makes the exercise easier. Flip the Ab Roller Evolution over so the bar and neck rest are on the floor and the curved handles are upright. Check that it is on a stable, flat surface and not on a movable rug or slippery floor—be certain it doesn't wobble!

Face toward the headrest and position your hands in the middle of the curved sides of the Ab Roller. Ease back on your toes, with your feet together, and extend your entire body. Your arms should be straight and your entire body balanced on your toes and hands, with the back straight from head to heels. Your body should form a 45-degree angle to the floor. Have a watch or big clock within eyesight to help keep track of timing your slower reps.

First Negative

Start to lower your body by bending your elbows. Focus on keeping your entire body straight. Don't let it sag.

Try to be halfway down at 10 seconds. At 15 seconds, your chest should be almost touching your hands. From the side, there's approximately a 90-degree bend in your elbows.

Positive

Start the positive pushing slowly, 1 inch by 1 inch. Try to be halfway up at 10 seconds.

Continue pushing with your arms and chest muscles. Check your body and make sure you are in a relatively rigid position. Extend your elbows completely at 15 seconds.

Second Negative

Repeat the procedure for the first negative. Try to be halfway down at 10 seconds and with your chest near your hands at 15 seconds.

Regular Reps

From the bottom position, immediately start regular-speed repetitions. Try for 8 to 12.

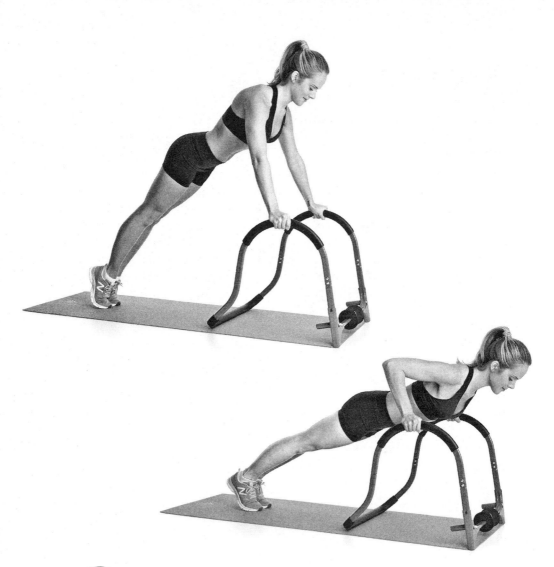

TIP • *After 15-15-15 negative-accentuated pushups, your regular reps will be very tough. You may want to rest for 30 seconds before starting regular repetitions. And it's okay if you do fewer than 8. But try to perform those you can do with good form.*

Adjust the toughness!

HARDER: ALLOW YOUR CHEST TO GO lower on each negative repetition. Increasing your range of motion this way makes the exercise more difficult.

Ab Roller Squat

MUSCLES WORKED: HAMSTRINGS, QUADRICEPS, AND GLUTEALS

Preparation

Flip the Ab Roller Evolution over so the bar and neck rest are on the floor and the curved handles are upright. Check that it is on a stable, flat surface and not on a movable rug or slippery floor—be certain it doesn't wobble!

Stand inside the unit with the headrest in front of you and your arms straight at your sides. Plant your feet shoulder-width apart, with your toes turned out slightly. Have a watch or big clock within eyesight to help keep track of timing your slower reps. If you need help rising from the squat position, place your hands on the sides of the Ab Roller.

First Negative

From a standing position, start bending your hips and knees slowly, inch by inch. Lower your buttocks smoothly, but keep your lower back slightly arched as you descend. You should be halfway down at 10 seconds.

Breathe as you keep lowering. If you feel insecure, move your hands near your hips so you can touch the sides of the Ab Roller for balancing.

Go as low as you can, without lifting your heels, to 15 seconds.

Positive

Push down through your heels, not your toes, as you inch your way up. You should feel an intense contraction in your thighs.

Keep your head and shoulders up and focus on your breathing. You should be halfway up at 10 seconds. Continue the slow ascent, standing erect at the 15-second mark.

Second Negative

Repeat the slow lowering from the first negative.

Focus, breathe, and keep your core rigid. You should be halfway down at 10 seconds. The hardest part is from halfway down to the bottom at 15 seconds.

Regular Reps

Push through your heels to rise and complete 8 to 12 normal-speed repetitions, taking 1 to 2 seconds for the positive and 2 seconds for the negative. Use the Ab Roller for help if you need it. The negative phase should take a little longer than the positive.

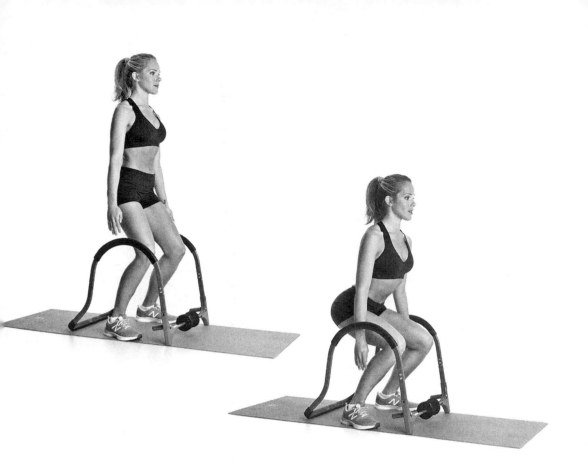

TIPS
- *Push your hips back as you near the bottom, but do not round your lower back. Keep your lower back slightly arched.*
- *Some people may have difficulty squatting below a level where the tops of their thighs are parallel to the floor. Others can almost touch their butt to their heels. See what feels most comfortable yet challenging for you. If your ankles are tight and you tend to lift your heels at the bottom of the squat, try placing a 1-inch board under your heels for stability.*

Adjust the toughness!

EASIER: USE THE AB ROLLER FOR support or do the negative-accentuated phase faster.

HARDER: SQUAT DEEPER, WHICH INCREASES YOUR range of motion.

Dumbbell Curl

MUSCLES WORKED: BICEPS

Preparation

Grasp a dumbbell in each hand and stand with your feet about shoulder-width apart. Most women feel comfortable starting with 5- or 10-pound dumbbells. As you stand, use some upward momentum and curl the weight to your shoulders. Anchor your elbows firmly against your sides. Keep a watch or big clock within eyesight to keep track of your timing on slow reps.

First Negative

Lower the dumbbells slowly, 1 inch by 1 inch. Reach the halfway-down position at 10 seconds.

Keep your torso erect as you reach the bottom position at 15 seconds.

Positive

From the bottom position, immediately begin curling the dumbbells up. Stabilize your elbows as you slowly lift the dumbbells to the halfway point at the 10-second mark.

Keep moving $\frac{1}{2}$ inch by $\frac{1}{2}$ inch. Pause in the top position at 15 seconds, but do not move your elbows forward. Keep them anchored against the sides of your waist.

Second Negative

Start the final descent and progress $\frac{1}{2}$ inch by $\frac{1}{2}$ inch. Be halfway down at 10 seconds.

Keep your elbows anchored firmly against your sides. Reach the bottom at 15 seconds.

Regular Reps

Perform 8 dumbbell curls smoothly at normal speed, taking 1 second for the positive and 2 seconds for the negative.

Push yourself and complete 8 repetitions. Place the dumbbells on the floor and relax.

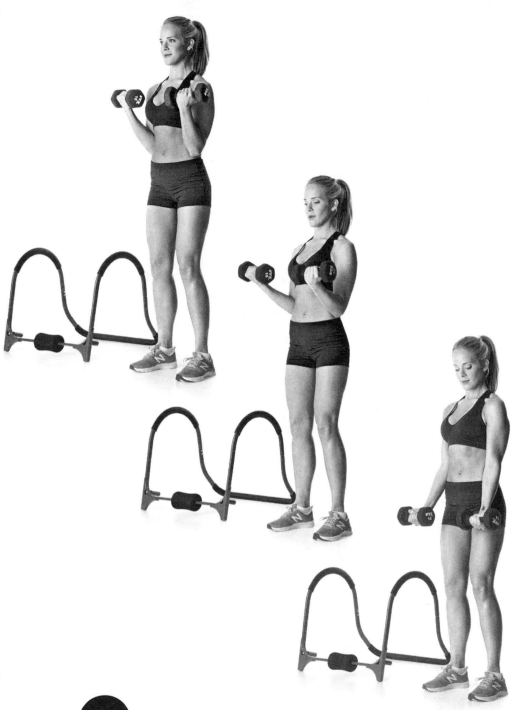

TIP • *Maximize your biceps stimulation by minimizing your body sway. Do not lean forward excessively or lean backward. Do not move your upper arms. Move only your hands, your forearms, and the dumbbells.*

Dumbbell Overhead Press

MUSCLES WORKED: DELTOIDS AND TRICEPS

Preparation

Choose a pair of light dumbbells. Five- to 10-pound dumbbells are ideal.

Place your feet shoulder-width apart, bend your knees slightly, and quickly press the dumbbells overhead. The dumbbells should be shoulder-width apart, and unlike a barbell that runs lengthwise across your shoulders, the dumbbells should be held parallel to each other, your palms facing each other. This is known as a neutral grip. Keep a watch or big clock within eyesight to keep track of your timing on slow reps.

First Negative

Lower the dumbbells slowly, inch by inch. Reach the halfway-down position at 10 seconds.

Keep the dumbbells apart and parallel to each other. Touch the dumbbells to your shoulders at 15 seconds.

Positive

Now press the dumbbells up slowly and smoothly, inch by inch. Be halfway up at 10 seconds.

Lock your elbows at 15 seconds. The dumbbells should still be parallel to each other.

Second Negative

Repeat the procedure for the first negative. Guide the dumbbells down slowly, inch by inch.

Move past the halfway point at 10 seconds. Touch the dumbbells to your shoulders at 15 seconds.

Regular Reps

Begin your regular-speed dumbbell presses smoothly, taking 1 second for the positive and 2 seconds for the negative. Try to complete 8 repetitions.

Place the dumbbells on the floor and relax.

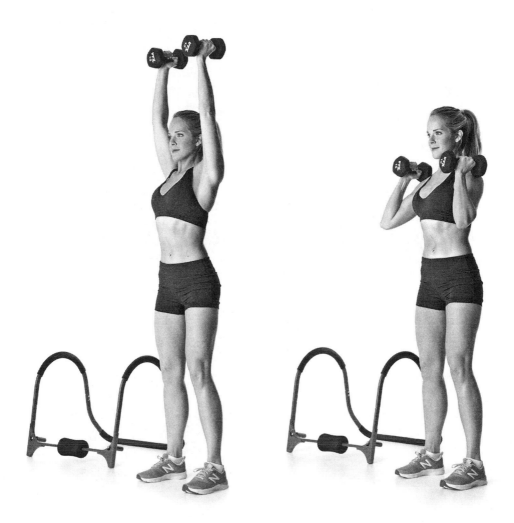

TIPS • *Keep your lower back naturally arched during the movements.*
• *It may take you several sessions to learn the mechanics of the negative-accentuated dumbbell overhead press, but it will be well worth it.*

BEFORE & AFTER 2 WEEKS

Pam Waters

Age 60 • Height 5 feet, 0.25 inch

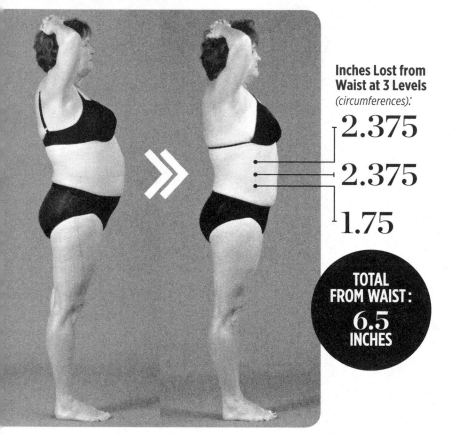

Inches Lost from Waist at 3 Levels *(circumferences):*

2.375

2.375

1.75

TOTAL FROM WAIST:

6.5 INCHES

Weight Before: **145.5 pounds**
Weight After: **135 pounds**
FAT LOSS: 11.61 pounds
Muscle Gain: **1.11 pounds**

"I can hardly believe the results. I went to bed early, to avoid snacking, and I got up after 8.5 hours and could actually feel my waist getting tighter each morning. I was snoozing and losing. What a great practice."

—*Pam Waters*

chapter

11

Snooze to Lose

The Importance of Extra Sleep

If you are trying to lose fat quickly, close your eyes and hum yourself a lullaby.

A number of recent studies have shown that getting high-quality sleep and maintaining a regular sleep routine correlate with lower body fat. One particular trial followed 245 overweight women ages 35 to 55 who were involved in a weight-loss program. The study's researchers reported in a 2012 issue of the journal *Obesity* that getting good-quality slumber and more than 7 hours of sleep per night increased the likelihood of weight-loss success by 33 percent.

Most people don't realize that at least 50 percent of the daily fat loss occurs while you are sleeping. That is especially true if you are on a 1,000-calorie-a-day eating plan combined with a rigorous exercise routine.

So, to make the entire Tighten Your Tummy program really work—especially for the first 2 weeks—I want you to do three important things in addition to the diet and exercise program:

- Get at least 8½ hours of sleep each night.

- Be less active throughout the day and night.

- Try to take a 30-minute afternoon nap.

What makes the above three guidelines so important—besides the fact that they worked like magic for my wife, Jeanenne, and most of the 41 women in the Tighten Your Tummy program in Gainesville—is that they are based on science. The primary scientific study that I'm referring to was reported by Dr. Arlet V. Nedeltcheva and colleagues in the *Annals of Internal Medicine* in 2010. The title of the study was "Insufficient Sleep Undermines Dietary Efforts to Reduce Adiposity." Let's take a close look at this research.

Sleep: One of the Most Powerful Fat-Loss Tools

This study compared two groups of overfat people who each ate 1,450 calories per day for 14 days. One group logged 8½ hours of sleep per night, and the other clocked 5½ hours per night (which the authors noted is the "norm" for most adults today). After 2 weeks, the people who slept longer lost significantly more fat than the group who slept less.

I know from my research that most dieters who do not strength-train end up losing both fat and muscle weight, and that's just what happened to both of the groups in Dr. Nedeltcheva's study. But get this: The sleep-deprived group dropped 60 percent more muscle than the group who slept more. Those 3 hours of missing sleep caused a shift in metabolism that made the body want to preserve fat at the expense of muscle. Remember, muscle burns more calories even at rest than fat does, so those unfortunate chronically tired folks had reduced the power of one of their bodies' key fat fighters.

That was not all. When the researchers compared circulating blood levels of appetite-regulating hormones in the two groups, they found that those who slept for 3 fewer hours produced more of the appetite-stimulating hormone *ghrelin*. In other words, when they woke up, they were hungrier.

Many people assume that their bodies burn more calories when they are awake longer, but that is not the case. Less sleep causes your metabolic rate to slow down. In other words, when you sleep less, your body starts to burn calories at a slower rate in an attempt to preserve energy.

Here's another significant finding: In the study, participants burned on average 400 more calories by sleeping for 3 more hours (for 8½ hours total). That's an additional 2,800 calories in one week or 5,600 calories for 2 weeks, which is very significant.

If that's not a great example of Snooze to Lose, what is?

With less sleep, the body seeks to meet the increased metabolic needs of longer waking hours by shifting into a lower gear that burns more muscle and less fat. That's exactly what you don't want to happen when your goal is losing weight and tightening your tummy!

In the final analysis, if you want to preserve muscle, burn fat, and wake up less hungry when you are dieting, sleep at least 8½ hours a night.

Inactivity: One of the Most Powerful Muscle-Building Tools

As I mentioned before, Arthur Jones is the man who invented Nautilus strength-training machines, which revolutionized the health club business in the 1970s and '80s. For 40 years, this pioneer of strength training explored the question, If a muscle is stimulated to grow, when does it actually grow? He could never boil it down to an exact time, but he did establish the following:

- Muscular growth, once it is stimulated, requires inactivity. To make sure you get stronger, firmer muscles from exercise, you must rest more, especially on the days in between workouts.

- More than 90 percent of muscular growth occurs during sleep and probably during a deep-sleep period of only 5 to 10 minutes.

- If in doubt about how much rest and sleep to get, err on the side of too much rather than too little.

During the research for my Body Fat Breakthrough program, I observed some revealing behaviors among participants in the negative-accentuated exercise program using the X-Force machines I mentioned in Chapter 5: After a particularly challenging workout, some of the men and women fell asleep on the floor of the fitness club's dressing room! I believe that this intense strength training caused greater muscle fatigue, which I call

TIPS FOR A BETTER NIGHT'S SLEEP

ESTABLISH A SCHEDULE. Your body craves routine. Go to bed at roughly the same time each night and wake at the same time. Even on weekends.

DON'T EAT HEAVY FOODS IN THE EVENING. A bloated belly may keep you from falling asleep.

AVOID CAFFEINE AFTER SUNSET. The stimulant can interfere with your ability to fall asleep. If you are caffeine sensitive, you may find that you have to stop drinking caffein-ated beverages (and even chocolate) earlier in the day, around 3 p.m.

AVOID ALCOHOL, TOO. You may think a glass of wine will make you tired, and it may do that, but it may also keep you from getting quality sleep.

TAKE A HOT BATH OR SHOWER BEFORE BED. Because sleep comes as the body's temperature drops, you can exaggerate the effect by warming your body, then cooling it by lying down under a sheet.

TURN OFF THE TV. Don't fall asleep to a TV show. And keep your bedroom pitch black. Even the smallest amount of light from a laptop, smartphone, or digital alarm clock can disturb your sleep.

KEEP YOUR BEDROOM COOL AND QUIET. Your body temperature naturally dips at night as part of preparation for sleep. Enhance that effect by turning your thermostat down. If your partner snores or teenagers are watching TV in the living room, drown out the noise with a tabletop fan or a sound machine that produces white noise.

"deeper inroad"—perhaps 40 to 50 percent deeper than normal training provides. This deeper inroad triggers the production of at least six hormones: growth hormone, insulin-like growth factor, mechano-growth factor, interleukin-6, interleukin-15, and insulin. The effects of these hormones on the human body were fatigue, rest, and deep sleep—and they all occurred quickly.

Note: I also observed the above happening to a lesser degree among the hardest-working Tighten Your Tummy women. They were snoozing more and losing more fat.

Naps Can Improve Your Results

Okay, so in addition to getting $8\frac{1}{2}$ hours of sleep each night, I'm now asking you to take an afternoon nap, right? Yes, that's correct. Here's why.

Cheri Mah, MS, a researcher at the Stanford Sleep Disorders Clinic and Research Laboratory, asked members of Stanford University's varsity basketball team in 2005 to try to sleep more. Every one of them did, and in doing so improved their performance in sprinting, free-throw shooting, and three-point shooting. Such findings eventually caught the attention of a number of NBA players, such as Steve Nash, Kobe Bryant, and LeBron James—all of whom slept more, liked it, and performed better. "Many athletes have optimized physical training and recovery," Mah said. "There really hasn't been the same emphasis on optimizing sleep and recovery."

The Stanford players and the initial NBA athletes were encouraged to nap every day. Even a brief nap can help the body release crucial growth hormones, which stimulate the healing of muscle and bone. Daily naps were like a magic pill to them.

Enter Charles Czeisler, MD, PhD, a professor at Harvard Medical School and today the go-to expert for professional sports teams from every major league. He noted that sleep deprivation could lead to high blood pressure, depression, and weight gain, as well as poor performance. What many athletes don't recognize is that it's the sleep after a game, or even after an intense workout, that's most important. Dr. Czeisler is convinced that a 30-minute midafternoon nap can do wonders for recovery. And that's precisely 30 minutes—no less and no more.

NAP LIKE A CAT

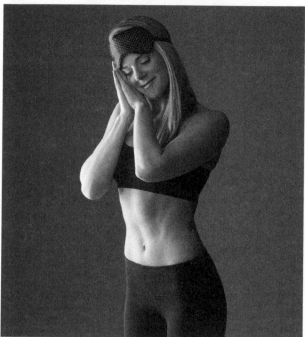

NEVER NAPPED? FOR SOME, IT TAKES a little effort. Setting the stage can make it easier to nod off. Here's how:

1. **TIME IT RIGHT.** Try for between 2 and 4 p.m., the time your circadian cycle dips. Napping later in the day may make it harder to fall asleep at night.

2. **SET AN ALARM.** Napping longer than 30 minutes may leave you groggy and disrupt nighttime sleep.

3. **NAP IN BED.** A cool, dark room will help you fall asleep quicker.

4. **DON'T HIT THE SNOOZE BUTTON.** When the alarm goes off, get right up. Walk around, splash some water on your face, do a few jumping jacks—anything to wake you up and make you active again.

I believe a midafternoon nap not only helps muscle recovery but also contributes to fat loss and tummy tightening. I've seen it happen in my wife and the many men and women who have participated in my fitness programs over the years.

Your Snooze Button for Losing Weight

After working with 145 people in the Body Fat Breakthrough program and 41 women in the Tighten Your Tummy program, my best advice for the first 14 consecutive days is as follows:

- Take a 30-minute nap each afternoon.

- Be less active during the day and night. Say no to vigorous activities.

- Go to bed an hour earlier each night, but get up at your normal time.

- Your goal is $8\frac{1}{2}$ hours of sleep each night. When you add in the naps, this equals 9 hours of sleep each 24 hours.

I strongly believe that adhering to these guidelines will help you achieve the fastest fat loss and tummy tightening possible. Practice Snooze to Lose faithfully and your belly will never be the same.

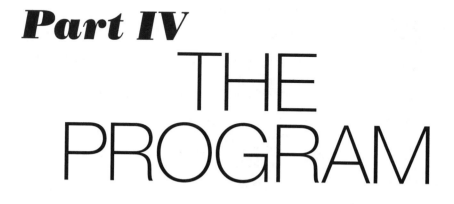

Part IV
THE
PROGRAM

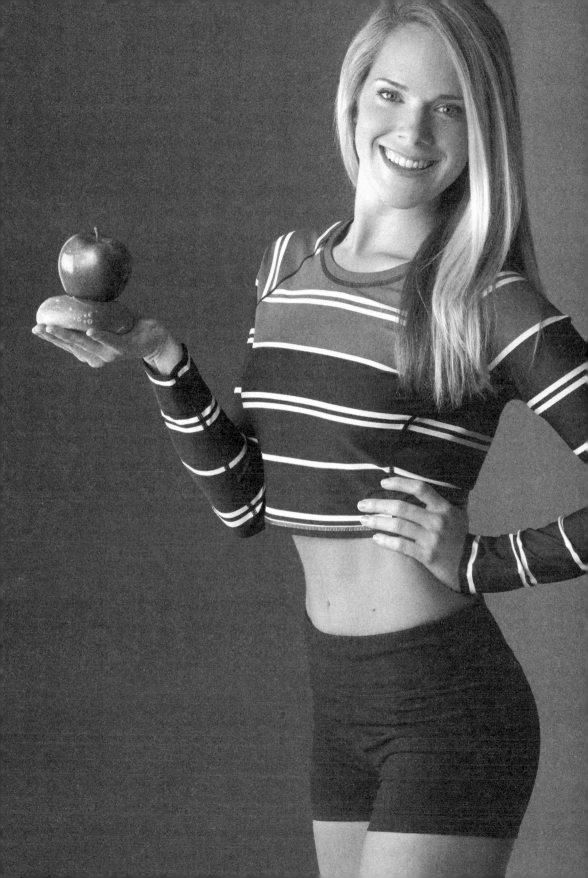

BEFORE & AFTER 6 WEEKS

Joan Cortez

Age 62 • Height 5 feet, 4.5 inches

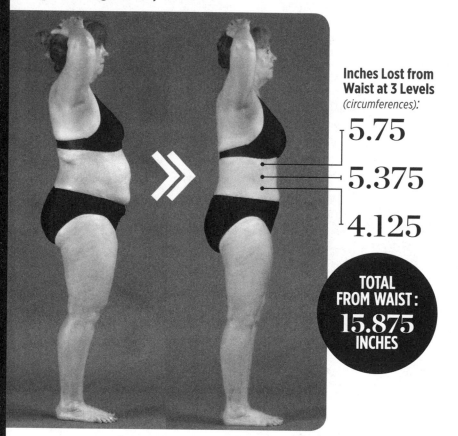

Inches Lost from Waist at 3 Levels
(circumferences):

5.75

5.375

4.125

TOTAL FROM WAIST :
15.875
INCHES

Weight Before: **197 pounds**
Weight After: **183 pounds**
FAT LOSS: 16.79 pounds
Muscle Gain: **2.79 pounds**

"What was once a huge mountain has now become a small hill. I have been given a second chance, and I am succeeding."

—Joan Cortez

chapter
12
What to Expect

After 2 Weeks and 6 Weeks

You're almost ready to start the Tighten Your Tummy program. But first, you would like to know what to expect—if you do commit—after 2 weeks, 6 weeks, and perhaps even 12 weeks?

The best way to answer your questions is to take a look at the test panel, how I organized the program, and overall averages of the women who progressed through each phase. You will be following a similar program and should expect similar results.

The Test Panel and the Organization

I recruited a test panel of 41 women from Gainesville Health & Fitness to go through the Tighten Your Tummy program in the fall of 2014. There was only one requirement: Each woman needed to lose at least 20 pounds of fat.

I weighed, measured, and photographed each participant on a Sunday and then introduced them to the program, handed out dietary informa-tion including a shopping list, discussed the exercise segments, and began the program on the following Monday morning. We conducted group exercise sessions twice a week, in the early afternoon. Each session lasted about 20 minutes or no longer than 30 minutes.

The twice-a-week exercise sessions were conducted in group style, with Pam Harrison, a personal trainer at the fitness center, leading the class. I was at each session, walking among the women, making sure the exercises were performed correctly. I taught the participants how to do each exercise using the negative-accentuated method—15-15-15, plus 8 to 12 repetitions—described in Chapter 10.

In addition to the twice-a-week exercise sessions, each woman did the following each day:

- Consumed 1,000 dietary calories

- Practiced the inner-ab vacuum twice before each meal

- Drank 1 gallon of ice water

- Walked for 30 minutes after the evening meal

- Slept 8½ hours at night

The program continued for three 2-week segments, with slight changes in each one. During Weeks 1 and 2, the participants kept calories to 1,000 a day and completed 1 set of five exercises. During Weeks 3 and 4, I increased the calories to 1,200 per day and added a new exercise to the workout. During Weeks 5 and 6, calories decreased to 1,100 a day, and we added another exercise to the routine. The other requirements—practicing the inner-ab vacuum, drinking ice water, walking after the evening meal, and sleeping 8½ hours per night—remained the same.

The program progressed smoothly, and all the women appeared moti-vated to do their best. Near the completion of Day 14, I asked the 21 women who were close to losing 10 pounds of body weight to allow me to measure and photograph them again on the next Sunday. I did so, and to my satisfac-tion, each one had lost more than 10 pounds of fat in only 14 days. A few of them dropped even more.

Results after 2 Weeks

The list below shows the 2014 test panel averages of 21 women who were measured after the first 2 weeks.

WOMEN (n = 21)

Averages

Age: 45.3 years

Height: 66.3 inches

Starting body weight:
163.7 pounds

Weight loss: 10.41 pounds

Fat loss: 12.72 pounds

Muscle gain: 2.31 pounds

Inches lost from waist:

2 inches above navel:
2.52 inches

At navel: 3.02 inches

2 inches below navel:
2.55 inches

Total of 3 measurements:
8.09 inches

An Interesting Comparison

In a similar study, which I published in 1992, 100 women from Gainesville Health & Fitness were also placed on a 1,000-calorie-a-day diet, combined with superhydration, but this group did not do negative-accentuated strength exercises. They did do conventional strength exercises in a group three times per week.

There was also another important difference: In 1992, I recruited women who needed to lose approximately 10 pounds of fat, not 20 or more pounds as in the 2014 study. Thus the average age, height, and starting body weight of these women was as follows: 33.44 years, 64.78 inches, and 134.76 pounds. The 1992 group was younger, shorter, and lighter. It's still interesting to examine and compare the outcomes.

The 1992 results: Of the 100 women, the average fat loss was 7.02 pounds, 1.83 inches off the waist (best of three measurement sites), plus a muscle gain of 1.26 pounds. Interestingly, only 7 of the 100 women lost 10 or more pounds of fat in 14 days.

The most pounds and inches that any of the 1992 women lost was 10.34 pounds of fat and 3.5 inches off the waist. Certainly, 3.5 inches off the waist in 2 weeks is very commendable. But in my 2014 group, one woman lost 5.5 inches off her waist at the below-navel level and 14.125 inches total from the combined three sites, again in only 2 weeks. The average inches lost from each of the three circumference sites were 2.5, 3, and 2.5—for a three-site total of 8 inches.

Furthermore, my 2014 group almost doubled (81 percent) the pounds lost of my 1992 group. The average fat loss of the 2014 group was 12.72 pounds versus 7.02 pounds for the earlier group. One of the 21 women from my 2014 group lost 15 pounds and four more lost 14 pounds of fat. That's an average of slightly more than 1 pound of fat a day for 14 consecutive days. And the muscle gain of the 2014 group (2.31 pounds to 1.26 pounds) was 83 percent better than the 1992 group. I've never had a group of female test panelists lose that much fat and gain that much muscle, period.

In my 1992 group, 7 of 100 lost 10 pounds of fat, which is a 7 percent success rate. In 2014, 21 of 41 women did, which is a success rate of 51 percent.

So if your goal is to lose 10 pounds of fat and significant inches off your waist in 2 weeks, then my 2014 Tighten Your Tummy program, compared to my 1992 plan, offers you a 700 percent better rate of success. And you'll only train twice a week versus three times a week for my 1992 group, which amounts to one-third less training time.

Results after 6 Weeks

Let's examine the average results of the 41 women who completed 6 weeks of Tighten Your Tummy training.

WOMEN (n = 41)

Averages

Age: 48.38 years

Height: 66.52 inches

Starting body weight: 164.14 pounds

Weight loss: 12.25 pounds

Fat loss: 15.28 pounds

Muscle gain: 3.03 pounds

Inches lost from waist:

2 inches above navel: 3.78 inches

At navel: 3.87 inches

2 inches below navel: 3.6 inches

Total of 3 measurements: 11.25 inches

Note: Of the 41 women finishing the program, six of them decided to go through a second time. Their 12-week results and averages will be discussed in Chapter 16.

Over 6 weeks, the top finisher was Roxanne Dybevick, 54, 5 feet 5 inches tall with a starting body weight of 164 pounds. Roxanne dropped 23.27 pounds of fat and built 5.97 pounds of muscle.

When I first met Roxanne, she had a quiet determination. But underneath that, I could see "the eye of a tiger." Sensing that she might do the best in the group, I asked her to keep a daily diary of the program. You can read her daily notes in Chapter 18.

"The Tighten Your Tummy program changed my life," Roxanne said. "I now feel back to my younger self . . . like a time machine whizzed me to 20 years earlier, when I was excited about life and all things were possible. I took all my fat-lady clothes to Goodwill, and I'm never looking back."

2 Weeks versus 6 Weeks

I usually recommend my 6-week programs to women. Most women who want to lose 10 pounds of fat need a full 6 weeks to learn, practice, and get the system to work in their favor. But the first 2 weeks of this program were different. They were remarkable in that they produced such amazing fat loss, inch loss, and muscle gain in only 14 days.

For example, the group of 21 women who were measured and photographed after 2 weeks, and then again after 6 weeks, had some revealing comparison numbers. After 6 weeks, the average fat loss per woman was 18.58 pounds. Looking at the earlier 2-week data revealed that on average, each woman lost 12.72 pounds of fat. That 12.72 pounds is disproportionately large compared to what I would normally expect from Weeks 1 and 2.

In fact, 12.72 pounds is 67 percent of the 6-week number of 18.58 pounds. In other words, these 21 women achieved approximately two-thirds of their fat loss during the first 2 weeks—which is a phenomenal result. That's almost 0.9 pound of fat loss per day for 14 consecutive days. I seriously doubt that anyone in the world has ever gotten such fantastic results from a group of 21 women in such a short period.

How did we achieve these amazing results? I believe four factors were most important.

- **15-15-15, plus 8 to 12 repetitions:** There's no doubt that this form of negative-accentuated training is superb. I watched in awe as the women trained more intensely, and with deeper inroads, than they had in the past. Many of them were changing right before my eyes. Furthermore, since I came up with this idea—in June 2014—I've personally trained 12 of my best clients with this technique once a week for 3 months or longer, with equally satisfying results.

- **Inner-ab vacuum:** I focused on teaching the inner-ab vacuum during the introductory meeting and the first training session, and all of the women got the hang of it quickly. Working the inner abs or transverse abdominis forced the women to be more conscious of their midsections, their feelings of fullness, and even their posture.

- **Extra sleep and rest:** Reread Chapter 11 and you'll see why getting $8\frac{1}{2}$ hours of sleep each night, plus a midafternoon nap, and plenty of inactivity during the day and night were critically important. I pushed these guidelines during each exercise session.

- **Group dynamics:** During my last 6-week program at Gainesville Health & Fitness, we had five women who were going through a second time. These five women acted as mentors to the first-time women, and that was helpful. Two of these mentors—Katie Smith, 60, and Joan Cortez, 62—were retired high school teachers who were instrumental in promoting a back-and-forth, open-door communication, not only among the test-panel women but also between them and me. Getting involved with other women who have similar fat-loss goals as you is a step in the right direction.

Of my test panel of 41 women, 5 of them lost 14 or more pounds of fat in 14 days:

- Roxanne Dybevick: 15.08 pounds

- Angela Choate: 14.8 pounds

- Katie Smith: 14.51 pounds

- Denise Rodriguez: 14.49 pounds

- Brianna Kramer: 14.26 pounds

And remember Sara Smith, whom I recognized in Chapter 2 for being number one in inches lost from the waist? Sara trimmed a total of 14.125 inches from her three waistline sites in just 14 days. Joan Cortez came in a close second at 13.5 total inches lost in 14 days.

Get ready for your transformation.

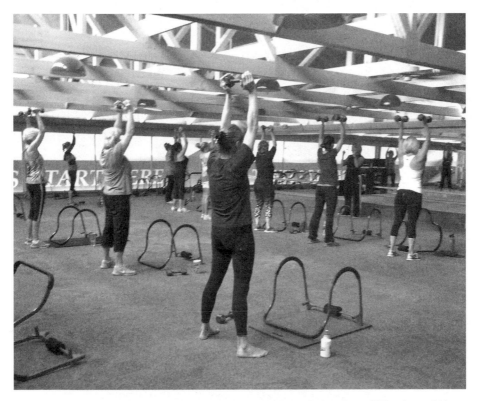

Gainesville test panelists perform the dumbbell overhead press. Remember, the lowering and lifting phases of this and other exercises require a slow 15 seconds down, 15 seconds up, and 15 seconds down movement followed by 8 to 12 faster reps.

BEFORE & AFTER 2 WEEKS

Amy Barber
Age 48 • Height 5 feet, 6 inches

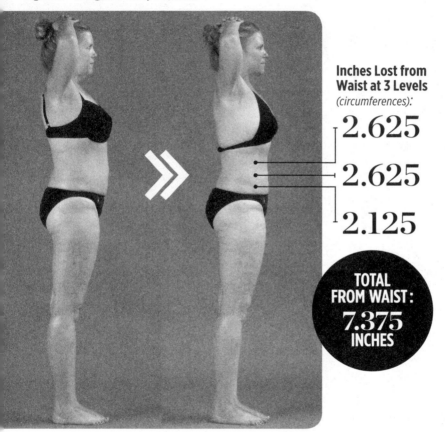

Inches Lost from Waist at 3 Levels
(circumferences):

2.625

2.625

2.125

TOTAL FROM WAIST: 7.375 INCHES

Weight Before: **156.7 pounds**
Weight After: **146.1 pounds**
FAT LOSS: 12.6 pounds
Muscle Gain: **2 pounds**

"Each day, I'm on the move. The program forced me to prepare. And preparation WORKS!"

—*Amy Barber*

chapter

13

Prepare to Succeed

10 Steps to Take before You Begin

Anything that is worth doing takes effort. There is no free lunch. Success requires work. I'm sure you've heard all that before. Well, I hope I haven't led you astray, because that's very true for the Tighten Your Tummy program, too.

Losing 14 pounds of fat in 14 days and achieving a tighter tummy is challenging. The program is remarkably effective, but no one can say it's supereasy. So don't expect to start this program and—wham, bish, bam—in 2 short weeks be showing off your well-defined abs in a bikini.

Sit up straight in your chair and listen to this reality check: It won't work without determination, discipline to follow the program exactly, and, most important, preparing to succeed. Every woman pictured in this book prepared to succeed.

"You have to prepare each day, and you have to follow up with sustained preparation," says Roxanne Dybevick, the test panelist who finished the 6-week program with the greatest overall results.

This chapter will help you do that. I think it's one of the most important in the entire book. So get out your pencil and paper or laptop—it's time to prepare to succeed. It all starts with the following 10 steps you need to take before beginning the Tighten Your Tummy program. Here they are.

1. Consult with Your Physician

Be sure your doctor knows you are going on the Tighten Your Tummy program. Let him examine this book so he understands what's involved. He may want to give you a physical if he hasn't given you one in the last year.

While this list isn't complete, certain people should not try this program: children and teenagers; women with certain types of heart, liver, or kidney disease; those with diabetes; and those suffering from some types of arthritis. Men shouldn't follow this program because the diet is too low in calories for most men. Some women should follow the program only with their physician's specific guidance and recommendations.

2. Recruit a Friend

Although it is certainly possible to get great results going through the program by yourself, you'll probably lose more pounds and inches if you team up with a friend or several friends. You and your friend should try to shop together, exercise together, walk together, and share each other's problems. Studies show that people who exercise together tend to stick with programs longer and achieve greater results because they motivate each other.

3. Take Measurements

You and your diet partner can best do the measurements together. In a private room, slip on your smallest bikini. A bikini works better than a one-piece bathing suit because it reveals your entire midsection. With a bathroom scale handy and a tape measure, record your "before," or starting, measurements in the chart on the opposite page. Fill in the other values at the end of the program.

	BEFORE	AFTER	DIFFERENCE
Body weight			
2″ above navel, belly relaxed			
At navel level, belly relaxed			
2″ below navel, belly relaxed			

Take all the measurements standing with your weight equally distributed on both feet. Apply the tape firmly, do not compress the skin, keep it parallel to the floor, and record the measurement to the nearest $1/8$ inch. You'll be taking circumference measurements at three levels: a high, a middle, and a low. Some women lose their fat at a greater or lesser degree from one or two of those levels, and you'll want to be aware of the differences.

4. Do the Pinch Test

You can get a fair estimate of your percent body fat by doing the pinch test.

The pinch test for women requires taking two measurements, the first one on the back of the upper arm and the second beside the navel. Here's the procedure to follow:

- Locate the first skin-fold site on the back of the right upper arm (triceps area) midway between the shoulder and elbow. Let the arm hang loosely at the side.

- Grasp a vertical fold of skin between the thumb and first finger. Pull the skin and fat away from the arm. Make sure the fold includes just skin and fat and no muscle.

- Use a ruler to measure the thickness of the skin to the nearest quarter of an inch. Be sure and measure the distance between the thumb and the finger. Sometimes the outer portion of the fold is thicker than the flesh grasped between the fingers. To avoid this, make sure the fold is level with the side of the thumb. Do not press the ruler against the skin. This will flatten it and make it appear thicker than it really is.

- Record two separate measurements of the triceps skin-fold thickness, releasing the skin between each measure, and calculate the average of the two.

- Locate the second skin-fold site, which is immediately adjacent to the right side of the navel.

- Grasp a vertical fold of skin between the thumb and first finger and follow the same technique as previously described.

- Record two separate measurements of the abdominal skin-fold thickness and calculate the average of the two.

- Add the average triceps skin-fold to the average abdominal skin-fold. This is your combined total.

- Estimate the percentage of body fat from the chart on the opposite page and record it on the chart below.

- Determine fat loss at the end of 6 weeks by multiplying percentage of body fat times body weight for the before-and-after tests. For example, if a woman weighed 168 pounds with 28 percent body fat at the start of the program, that's 47.04 pounds of fat. If she completed the program at 150 pounds and 18 percent body fat, that's 27 pounds of fat. The difference between 47.04 and 27 is 20.04 pounds.

- Figure the amount of muscle gain by subtracting the weight loss from the fat loss. In the example above, where fat loss equaled 20.04 pounds and weight loss was 18 pounds, 2.04 pounds of muscle were gained.

More than 25 percent of the body weight of most Americans is composed of fat. An ideal amount of body fat for most men is 12 percent. The average young woman's ideal status is 18 percent. Lean, athletic men and women may desire to lower their ideal figures by another 5 or 6 percentage points.

Pinch Test Measurements

	BEFORE	AFTER
Right triceps		
Right abdominal		
Total		
Body fat percent		
Fat pounds		

Estimated Percentage of Body Fat

SKIN-FOLD THICKNESS	PERCENT FAT	PERCENT FAT
TRICEPS PLUS ABDOMINAL	MEN	WOMEN
$^3/_4$ inch	5–9	8–13
1 inch	9–13	13–18
$1^1/_4$ inches	13–18	18–23
$1^1/_2$ inches	18–22	23–28
$1^3/_4$ inches	22–27	28–33
$2^1/_4$ inches	27–32	33–38
$2^3/_4$ inches	32–37	38–43

5. Take Full-Body Photographs

There is no better way to evaluate your current condition than to have full-body photographs taken of yourself in a bikini. Digital cameras are easy to use. Here are the best procedures to follow:

- Wear a solid-color bikini.

- Stand against an uncluttered, light-colored background.

- Direct the person with the camera to move away from you until your entire body is visible in the viewfinder. It's best for that person to be 15 to 20 feet from you and zoom in with the camera lens. The camera should be turned sideways for a vertical format. It's also best for the photographer to be seated with the camera approximately 3 feet off the floor.

- Stand relaxed for two pictures: front and right side. Do not try to suck in your stomach.

- Interlace your fingers and place them on top of your head, so the contours of your torso will be plainly visible. Keep your feet 8 inches apart for the front and back shots, but together on the side picture.

- Download the digital "before" photos onto your computer. Crop the best ones tightly into a 3-inch-by-6-inch size.

- Retake the photos 6 weeks later, following the same directions, with the same bathing suit and camera.

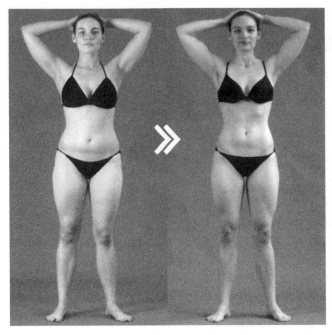

For the best before-and-after comparisons, you must standardize both sets of photos. Make the height and poses identical. Crop the photos exactly the same. Brianna Kramer, at left, dropped 20.86 pounds of fat and tightened her tummy by 9.875 inches in 6 weeks.

- Download your "after" images onto your computer.

- Crop and make the prints the same size as the "before" ones. Your height in both sets of photos should be precisely the same.

6. Visit Your Favorite Supermarket

The 2-week and 6-week eating plans in this book are the simplest I've ever designed. They also require the least amount of preparation. Furthermore, all the foods can be purchased from almost any large supermarket. You will, however, need to become well acquainted with certain sections of the store.

7. Use Measuring Spoons, Cups, and a Small Scale

Most people overestimate one-half cup of orange juice, one tablespoon of raisins, or one ounce of mozzarella cheese. Such practices lead to inaccurate calorie counting and inefficient fat loss. It is important to become familiar with and correctly use measuring spoons, cups, and food scales.

These items can be purchased inexpensively at your local department store or supermarket. With food scales, however, you'd be well advised to spend more money on a battery-operated, digital scale instead of the less expensive, spring-loaded type.

8. Take a Vitamin-Mineral Pill Each Day

You should take one multiple-vitamin-with-minerals tablet each morning while you are eating a reduced-calorie diet. The tablet should contain calcium and iron. Study the label, however, and make sure that no nutrient exceeds 100 percent of the Recommended Dietary Allowance. High-potency supplements and super-stress formulas are a waste of money.

9. Examine the Menus, Recipes, and Shopping Lists

Glance through the Tighten Your Tummy menus, recipes, and shopping lists in Chapters 14 and 15 for an overview of what you'll be eating during the 2-week and 6-week programs. Your results will be better if you plan ahead.

10. Get Serious

You've done your tests and measurements, and you've made certain purchases. Plus, you've familiarized yourself with what to expect. Now it's time to get serious. Sit quietly and think about your goals. Visualize success. Give yourself a pep talk if it helps. It's time to lose significant pounds and inches and tighten your tummy.

BEFORE & AFTER 2 WEEKS

Yu Yang
Age 46 • Height 5 feet, 7.5 inches

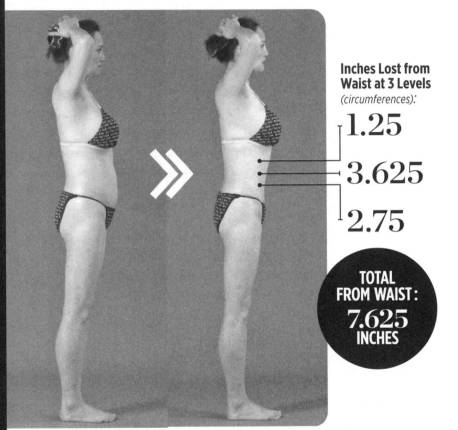

**Inches Lost from
Waist at 3 Levels**
(circumferences):

1.25

3.625

2.75

**TOTAL
FROM WAIST:**
7.625
INCHES

Weight Before: **137.9 pounds**
Weight After: **128.9 pounds**
FAT LOSS: 10.3 pounds
Muscle Gain: **1.3 pounds**

"The Power-Start
Diet made me feel
powerful . . . and
I like that feeling."
—*Yu Yang*

chapter
14
The Power-Start Diet

Simplify Your Meals in Weeks 1 and 2 for Automatic Success

The beauty of the Tighten Your Tummy diet is its acceptance of carbohydrates as your body's preferred fuel and the sheer simplicity of the eating plan. Several of the test panelists told me, "For 2 weeks, it took almost all the thinking out of dieting. You purchase a few foods and lock into the daily routine."

It's just that simple.

I've found that diets that are complicated and require time-consuming food shopping and preparation are difficult to maintain. That's why for the first 2 weeks especially, I recommend that you avoid variety, repeat meals you really like, and use frozen microwaveable meals for dinners to automate calorie and portion control.

I call the first 2 weeks of this program the Power-Start Diet because its quick, measurable results make dieters feel real, positive power:

- *Power* because they have built muscle at the same time they are losing fat

- *Power* because they definitely feel leaner and stronger

- *Power* because they are now ready to follow through, if necessary, with Weeks 3 through 6

- *Power* because that's what women want in their personal and professional lives—the confidence and powerful motivation that comes from achievement

Limit Your Choices

I've made every attempt to use current, popular brand names and calorie counts, which are listed in the menus. But as you probably know, products are frequently changed, modified, and discontinued. If a listed food choice is not available in your area for whatever reason, you'll have to substitute something similar. Become a label reader at your supermarket.

Thanks to the Web, it's easy to instantly check around town for availability of certain food products. Also, women doing the same program can share where they located hard-to-find food choices.

Each day, you will choose a limited selection of foods for breakfast and lunch. I've found that women can consume the same basic breakfast and lunch for months, with little or no modification. Ample variety during your evening meal, however, will make daily eating interesting and enjoyable. The eating plan includes snacks to keep your energy high and your hunger low.

Noncaloric beverages are any type of water—tap, bottled, carbonated, or flavored—with no calories. Other noncaloric beverages are soft drinks with zero calories.

For the latest frozen, microwaveable meals, and for possible dinner substitutions, refer to the following Web sites: Leancuisine.com, Michelinas. com, and Healthychoice.com. Don't forget you can also steam or microwave bags of vegetables and pair them with fresh proteins like fish, chicken, or lean beef to make mealtime easier.

Begin Week 1 on Monday and continue through Sunday. Week 2 is a repeat of Week 1. Calories for each food are noted in parentheses. A shopping list follows at the end of the chapter.

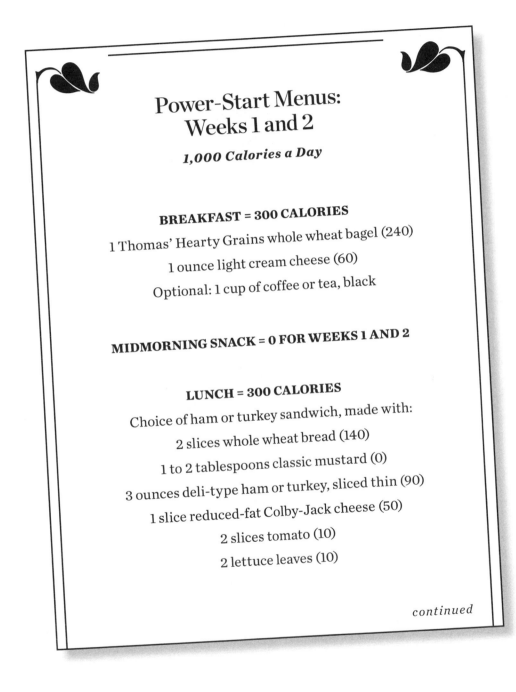

Power-Start Menus: Weeks 1 and 2

1,000 Calories a Day

BREAKFAST = 300 CALORIES

1 Thomas' Hearty Grains whole wheat bagel (240)

1 ounce light cream cheese (60)

Optional: 1 cup of coffee or tea, black

MIDMORNING SNACK = 0 FOR WEEKS 1 AND 2

LUNCH = 300 CALORIES

Choice of ham or turkey sandwich, made with:

2 slices whole wheat bread (140)

1 to 2 tablespoons classic mustard (0)

3 ounces deli-type ham or turkey, sliced thin (90)

1 slice reduced-fat Colby-Jack cheese (50)

2 slices tomato (10)

2 lettuce leaves (10)

continued

Power-Start Menus:
Weeks 1 and 2
continued

MIDAFTERNOON SNACK = 50 CALORIES

Choice of ½ apple, 3-inch diameter (50); 2 prunes; or ½ cup light or fat-free flavored yogurt (50)

DINNER = 300 CALORIES

Choose one of these frozen, microwaveable meals and a noncaloric beverage.

Orange Chicken, Lean Cuisine Culinary Collection (310)
Lemon Pepper Fish, Lean Cuisine Culinary Collection (300)
Three Cheese Ziti Marinara, Michelina's Lean Gourmet (300)

EVENING SNACK = 50 CALORIES

Choice of nuts: 7 whole unsalted almonds or cashews

OTHER DAILY GUIDELINES:

Drink 1 gallon (128 ounces) of ice-cold water.

Practice doing an inner-ab vacuum twice before each major meal.

Walk after dinner for 30 minutes.

Take a 30-minute nap in the afternoon if possible.

Go to bed an hour early and sleep 8½ hours.

Do the negative-accentuated exercise routine twice a week.

Shopping List for Weeks 1 and 2 Menus

The quantities for 1 week of the listed foods will depend on your specific selections. Review your choices and adjust the shopping list accordingly. Remember to check nutrition information on products you buy so that you can carefully follow the serving sizes in the menus. It may be helpful for you to photocopy this list each week before doing your shopping.

STAPLES

☐ Mustard

☐ Whole, unsalted almonds

☐ Whole, unsalted cashews

☐ Noncaloric beverages: bottled water, diet soft drinks, tea, and coffee

GRAINS

☐ Thomas' Hearty Grains whole wheat bagels

☐ Whole wheat bread

FRUITS

☐ Apples (3-inch diameter)

☐ Prunes

VEGETABLES

☐ Lettuce

☐ Tomatoes

DAIRY

☐ Light cream cheese

☐ Reduced-fat Colby-Jack cheese

☐ Light or fat-free flavored yogurt

MEAT AND ENTRÉES

☐ White turkey meat, thin sliced

☐ Ham, thin sliced

☐ Frozen, microwaveable dinners or entrées:

- *Orange Chicken, Lean Cuisine Culinary Collection*
- *Lemon Pepper Fish, Lean Cuisine Culinary Collection*
- *Three Cheese Ziti Marinara, Michelina's Lean Gourmet*

BEFORE & AFTER 6 WEEKS

Mary Dees
Age 61 • Height 5 feet, 4.5 inches

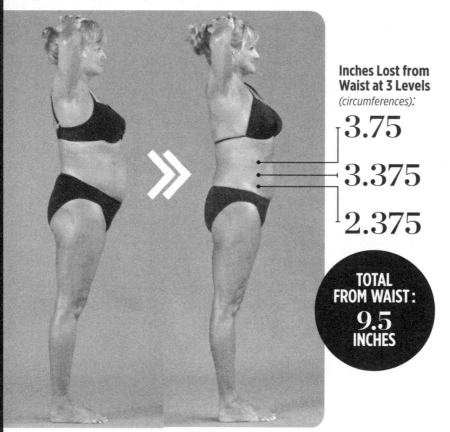

Inches Lost from Waist at 3 Levels *(circumferences):*

3.75

3.375

2.375

TOTAL FROM WAIST:
9.5
INCHES

Weight Before: **157.6 pounds**
Weight After: **142.75 pounds**
FAT LOSS: 17.75 pounds
Muscle Gain: **2.9 pounds**

"Dr. D opened my eyes to having a plan, sticking with it, and learning to say NO!"
—*Mary Dees*

chapter
15

How to Eat for Weeks 3–6

Don't Stop! There's More to Eat . . . and to Lose!

Have you reached your goal in just 2 weeks? A few women from the Gainesville test panel did just that and then stopped. Most of the women, however, continued for Weeks 3, 4, 5, and 6. You'll most likely want to keep going, so this chapter is devoted to the eating plan for the next 4 weeks.

After limited foods for Weeks 1 and 2, you'll welcome some variety and substitutions that are now available. Weeks 3 and 4 increase daily calories by 200, bringing you up to 1,200 per day. During Weeks 5 and 6, you will drop to 1,100 per day. This up-and-down concept seems to keep the body's energy system primed for efficient fat loss.

Here's the way the plan works.

WEEKS 3 AND 4: CONSUME 1,200 CALORIES A DAY

- Add 50 calories to midmorning snack: 7 whole unsalted almonds or cashews.

- Add 100 calories to midafternoon snack: more apple, prunes, or yogurt.

- Add 50 calories to evening snack: more nuts, prunes, or yogurt.

WEEKS 5 AND 6: CONSUME 1,100 CALORIES A DAY

- Remove 100 calories from midafternoon snack.

This may be substituted for a 300-calorie breakfast:

GoLean Cereal (285 calories)

> 1 cup Kashi GoLean Cereal (140)
> ½ cup fat-free milk (45) or 1 cup almond milk (45)
> 1 large banana (8¾" long) (100)

This may be substituted for a 300-calorie breakfast or lunch:

Meal Replacement Shake (300–320 calories)

> 2 scoops Metabolic Drive shake mix* (220) or 4 scoops EAS Lean 15 Protein Powder* (200)
> 1 large banana (8¾" long) (100)
> 8–12 ounces cold water

Place the ingredients in a blender and mix until smooth.

Learn more about these products at MetabolicDrive.com and EAS.com.

One of the following may be substituted for a 100-calorie snack:

- **An energy bar.** Popular bars—such as ZonePerfect, PowerBar, Odwalla, and Clif—may be used as snacks. Their calories range from 210 to 240, so eat only ½ bar.

Chef Salad (306 calories)

      2 cups chopped lettuce (20)

      2 ounces white meat, chicken or turkey (80)

      2 slices reduced-fat Colby-Jack cheese (100)

      4 slices tomato, chopped (28)

      1 tablespoon fat-free dressing (8)

      1 slice whole wheat bread, toasted and cut into cubes (70)

In a large bowl, mix the ingredients together.

Sandwich from Subway (300 calories)

- 6" Turkey Breast and Black Forest Ham on 9-Grain Wheat bread with plenty of raw vegetables; no oil-based dressings, only mustard

Tuna Salad (260 calories)

      ½ can (2.5 ounces) chunk light water-packed tuna (50)

      ½ cup (4 ounces) canned whole kernel corn, no salt added (60)

      ½ cup (4 ounces) canned sweet peas (60)

      2 tablespoons sweet pickle relish (40)

      1 tablespoon Hellmann's Light Mayonnaise (50)

      1 tablespoon Dijon mustard (0)

In a large bowl, mix the ingredients together.

- Santa Fe-Style Rice & Beans, Lean Cuisine Simple Favorites (290)
- Butternut Squash Ravioli, Lean Cuisine Spa Collection (260)
- Vegetable Egg Roll, Lean Cuisine Simple Favorites (300)
- Pineapple Black Pepper Beef, Lean Cuisine Honestly Good (320)

BEFORE & AFTER 18 WEEKS

Katie Smith
Age 60 • Height 5 feet, 4.75 inches

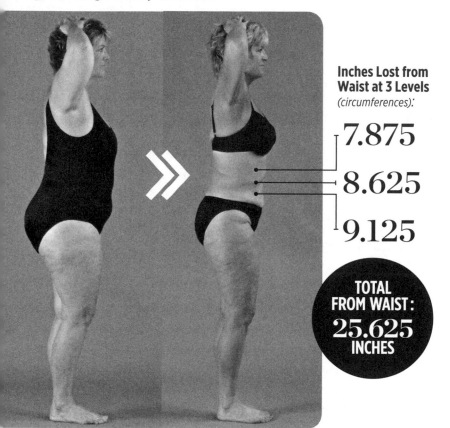

Inches Lost from Waist at 3 Levels *(circumferences):*

7.875

8.625

9.125

TOTAL FROM WAIST: 25.625 INCHES

Weight Before: **207.6 pounds**

Weight After: **152.1 pounds**

FAT LOSS: 62.73 pounds

Muscle Gain: **7.23 pounds**

"Being rained on is a wonderful metaphor for setbacks. I've had some in my life. But thanks to this program, my point of view is now supported by strength."

—*Katie Smith*

chapter

16

For Those Who Want More

An Optional Program for Extra Fat Loss

If you had more than 25 pounds of fat to lose when you started the 6-week Tighten Your Tummy program, then you probably need to repeat the course to reach your goal. But it will be even easier this time around because you're a pro!

Of the 41 women who finished the first 6 weeks, 6 decided to continue for a second time. All 6 had more than 25 pounds of fat to lose. Their average results are listed on the following page.

Results after 12 Weeks

WOMEN (n = 6)

Averages

Age: 48.33 years

Height: 65.94 inches

Starting body weight:
188.3 pounds

Weight loss: 24.4 pounds

Fat loss: 29.98 pounds

Muscle gain: 5.58 pounds

Inches lost from waist:

2 inches above navel:
5.6 inches

At navel: 5.19 inches

2 inches below navel:
4.625 inches

Total of 3 measurements:
15.415 inches

A Mother-and-Daughter Team

The test panelist who lost the most fat after 12 weeks was Katie Smith, age 60. Katie dropped 43.47 pounds of fat and built 8.82 pounds of muscle. Her 34-year-old daughter, Jennifer MacCallum, who also completed 12 weeks, finished as a runner-up by losing 34.07 pounds of fat. Get this: Katie and Jennifer each have four children! And they shed a combined 77.54 pounds. I guarantee you that their lives are now drastically improved.

"For 27 years, I've weighed over 200 pounds," Katie told the test group during their final weigh-in. "I had almost given up hope of ever returning to a somewhat normal body weight. Now look at me. I weigh 170 pounds and my goal is now to get down to 150 pounds. Nothing's going to stop me!" And it didn't. Katie continued for another 6 weeks and you've already seen her 18-week results on page 152.

Jennifer said, "I am so happy that I have some femininity sprinkled back into my figure. I have a curve in my lower back right above my jeans that makes me look much more shapely. I now have cheekbones and no double chin. When I'm blow-drying my hair, I notice in the mirror that my forearms look half the size."

Both of these remarkable women received a standing ovation from their friends.

Repeating the Program: Some Tips

There's magic in repeating what has already produced outstanding results. The six women who went through the test program a second time did not change a thing. They started their eating plan at 1,000 calories a day for Weeks 7 and 8, increased the calories to 1,200 for Weeks 9 and 10, and then decreased to 1,100 calories a day for Weeks 11 and 12.

Katie Smith, who lost 21.43 pounds over the first 6 weeks, lost 22.04 pounds during the second 6 weeks. It's unusual to have more fat loss during the second 6 weeks. I tell my test groups that repeat a program to expect to lose—under the best conditions—approximately 60 percent of the fat they dropped the first time. Katie's focused attitude paid big dividends in her repeated run.

A menu item that one of my repeats, Joan Cortez, recommended to her five teammates was a new frozen microwaveable dinner called SELF Healthy Kitchen. The ones we tested in Gainesville were all tasty and in the 300-calorie range. The following choices may be added to your evening meal selections:

- SELF Garden Chicken Alfredo (320)

- SELF Steak with Portobello Mushroom (280)

- SELF Southwest Style Beef Enchilada (310)

One of my repeating panelists pointed out that she preferred to limit the variety of her meal selections because it simplified her approach to disciplined eating.

That reminds me of a 2012 conversation I had with my best subject from the Body Fat Breakthrough program, Angel Rodriguez. Angel, who was severely obese at almost 50 percent body fat when he started that program, lost 121 pounds of fat by going through five back-to-back 6-week programs. I was curious as to how often Angel had substituted other options for the four Lean Cuisine-type microwaveable meals listed in the first 6-week eating plan. I asked him that question after he'd been on the diet for 30 weeks.

"What do you mean by substitutions?" Angel asked.

"You know, the additional menu items that I listed on the handout under the heading of 'Substitutions' some 28 weeks ago?"

"Substitutions? I don't remember there ever being any," he said, shaking his head. "So I never made any. I just keep repeating the same menus from Weeks 1 and 2 for the entire 30 weeks. They worked great for me."

"Great" is an understatement. Angel had locked into a menu that simplified his eating to only one page. There were no choices, nothing to think about. Just buy, open, cook or not cook, eat, and repeat—meal after meal, day after day, until all the excessive fat was removed. For Angel, that took exactly 210 days.

Simple. It worked for Angel. And it's an option for you.

Making It through the Rain

Let me tell you one final story about the mom-and-daughter team. Katie and Jennifer have beautiful voices and love to sing. They asked if they could sing at the celebration event at the end of the final Tighten Your Tummy program. I suggested a favorite song of mine that I thought would have relevance to them and the entire group. And they agreed.

A little background about the song: In 1984, I was working on a book

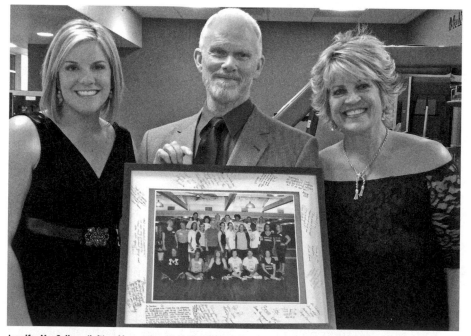

Jennifer MacCallum *(left)* and her mother, Katie Smith, present me with a Tighten Your Tummy Group 2 team photo, signed by all the members of the second test panel at our post-program celebration at Gainesville Health & Fitness.

project with a graphic designer for Putnam Publishing in New York City. Late one afternoon, I went to Times Square to get a half-price ticket for a Broadway musical. None of the plays I wanted to see had tickets available, so I settled for the Barry Manilow concert. I grew up in the 1950s, and ballads and soft tunes were my favorite types of music. I figured Manilow would be to my liking.

I was right. Manilow put on a great show. During his curtain call, he dedicated his final song, "I Made It Through the Rain," to anyone in the audience who had ever been picked on, laughed at, or told a hoped-for dream could not come true. "Losers can be winners," he said. I thought to myself, "Someday, I'm going to incorporate that story and his song into one of my presentations." And I found my opportunity during the Tighten Your Tummy program celebration.

Katie and Jennifer harmonized perfectly for the group and put their hearts into the lyrics:

When friends are hard to find

And life seems so unkind

Sometimes you feel afraid

Just aim beyond the clouds

And rise above the crowds

And start your own parade

Katie and Jennifer did just that the second time they went through the Tighten Your Tummy program. They became mentors to the new group of participants and succeeded beyond my dreams.

"We made it through the rain," they sang.

And so can you!

Part V
MAINTENANCE AND INSPIRATION

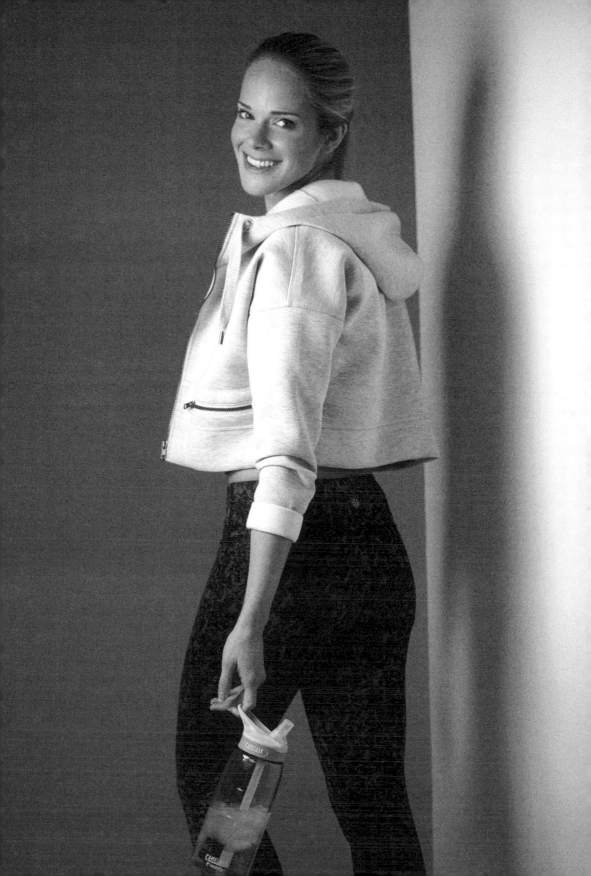

chapter
17

How to Keep Your New Look

Maintaining Your Tighter Tummy

Don't skip this chapter. It's important if you like your new body and want to keep it! If you haven't already noticed something a little different about how some of your friends are acting around you, then be prepared. Because sooner or later, you will.

They'll usually be very subtle about it. They'll offer you foods, often presented as gifts that go against your eating plan. Then they'll try to disrupt your exercise routine by asking you to meet them at the mall. Or they'll tease you about your ever-present water bottle. They may actually encourage you to be discouraged. Some may even express frustrations, suggesting that your positive behaviors are affecting their lives.

I've seen it happen numerous times. When a woman decides to lose fat, and is successful, she'll be surrounded by people trying to distract, disrupt, and even sabotage her.

Action always offends the inactive.

If you were raised in Texas near the Gulf of Mexico coastline as I was, then you may have heard this story about the blue-claw crabs. It's worth sharing.

The Crabs in a Tub Story

The blue crab, the delicious seafood that is easy to catch but difficult to clean, is prevalent along the Gulf Coast and also up and down the eastern coast of the United States.

I've been to many crab boils over the years. Before the crabs were cooked in big pots on the stove, about 20 of them, still alive, would be spread among several metal washtubs. Some of the hungry crowd, including me, would be watching the crabs inside the tubs.

Initially, to avoid becoming dinner, one or two crabs would try to escape by climbing on the backs of the others and then clawing their way up the sides of the container. If they employed a little teamwork, they could climb out. But guess what happened? The other crabs would reach up and pull the escaping crab back to the bottom of the tub. They did this repeatedly to each maverick that ventured up the metal wall.

The end result was that no crab escaped. Not one got out alive. All the crabs would eventually be cooked for a tasty meal.

That's what I believed. Then one time, I watched a single crab climb out of a tub. It happened so fast and so unexpectedly that I almost didn't notice. Then, within 30 seconds, another crab and another and another, in rapid order, made their escape from the same tub.

As I told others to come see the crabs stacking on top of one another and easily flopping over the edge, an older man, who was experienced in catching and cooking crabs, said to me, "Blue crabs are followers. One by one, they'll all lock on to the same bait for easy catching. Marooned in a tub, they see no cooperation, other than pinching and pulling any crab that tries to climb out. But once in a great while, you'll see them do this. I've seen it only a few times in 10 years."

Then the old man said something very interesting: "Crabs communicate mostly by sight. If you took slow-motion pictures as the first crab mounted the top edge of the tub and went over, you'd see a shot of him turning back slightly and pincer-waving for the others . . . to follow. You know, sort of like John Wayne did at the end of *Sands of Iwo Jima*?"

Crabs, once they see a strong tub mate achieving possible freedom, can not only follow but also learn how to lead. At least, a few can.

Be the Blue Crab That Escapes!

When you set a new physical goal—such as losing fat and building muscle—you have intentionally pointed out (whether you realize it or not) other people's weaknesses. You've hit them head-on with their lack of desire and inability to plan and prepare for improving their body. These people sit around and want. Your success angers them, and they'll try to pull you back to the bottom of the tub.

It's up to you to escape their grip. Don't spend a second of time worrying about the caged-in crabs. Tell them no, and mean it. Wriggle away from them—offend them, if necessary. You have worked hard for your success. Don't let anyone take it away from you. Remember, action offends the inactive. And that's their problem, not yours.

Here's another approach: Use your significantly stronger muscles to your advantage. You crawled out of the tub more than 6 weeks ago. Some of your friends, no doubt, are ready to follow you. Give them a chance, maybe even a second or third chance. Maybe it's time for you to become a mentor to friends who are ready to follow your lead to a tighter tummy.

Apply the Mechanics for Maintenance

Now that you've tasted success, you don't want to give up your tighter tummy and sleek new body. Your goal now is to maintain your ideal body weight, percent body fat, and waistline size. The secret to maintenance is in the mechanics—the mechanics of successful dieting and the mechanics of successful exercising.

Let's summarize what you have done to date to get to your new body:

- Focus on improving your muscle/fat ratio by building muscle and losing fat simultaneously.

- Keep your daily calories in the approximate range of 50 percent carbohydrates, 25 percent fats, and 25 percent proteins. The menus in this book are designed to do this for you.

- Vary your daily calories gradually with each 2-week period from 1,000 to 1,200 to 1,100.

- Drink 1 gallon of ice water each day.

- Exercise in a negative-accentuated style progressively twice a week.

- Look for ways to make your exercise harder, not easier.

- Take a 30-minute nap each day.

- Sleep 8½ hours each night.

- Practice being less active, rather than more active, each day.

On the Tighten Your Tummy maintenance plan, you must still watch how many calories you eat each day. Only now, rather than trying to lose fat, you're trying to maintain your weight and avoid putting fat back on. Most women can maintain their existing level of fat on 1,500 to 2,000 calories a day. There is no simple method to determine in advance how many calories you will need to maintain your weight. Trial and error is the obvious course of action. Let's begin by examining the maintenance chart on page 164.

To figure out your maintenance level, gradually add calories from the basic food groups—meat, milk, fruits/vegetables, breads/cereals, and other—to the 1,200 calorie-a-day diet you are already familiar with.

For example, try a certain level—say 1,600 calories a day—for 2 weeks. If your weight on the scale is still going down slightly, then raise your level to 1,800 a day for another 2 weeks. Your body weight should stabilize. Now you have reached the upper limit of your maintenance calorie level. It should not take you longer than a month to figure out your daily requirement for calories.

Maintenance Guidelines for Calories

FOOD	1,500	1,600	1,700	1,800	1,900	2,000
Meat Group	3 servings or total of 7 oz cooked	3 servings or total of 7 oz cooked	3 servings or total of 7 oz cooked	3+ servings or total of 8 oz cooked	3+ servings or total of 9 oz cooked	4 servings or total of 10 oz cooked
Milk Group	1 cup fat-free milk	2 cups fat-free milk	2 cups fat-free milk	2 cups fat-free milk	2 cups fat-free milk	2 cups fat-free milk
	1 cup whole milk	1 cup whole milk	1 cup whole milk	1 cup whole milk	1 cup whole milk	1 cup whole milk
Fruits and Vegetables Group	4 servings	4.5 servings	5 servings	5.5 servings	6 servings	6 servings
Breads and Cereals Group	5 servings	6 servings	6 servings	6 servings	6 servings	6 servings
Other	3 servings	3 servings	3 servings	3 servings	3 servings	3 servings

Meat Group: Choose lean, well-trimmed meats. Beef, veal, lamb, pork, poultry, and fish should have skin removed. One egg can be substituted for 1 serving of meat. One cup dried beans or peas can be substituted for 1 serving of meat. One ounce lean meat = 60 calories.

Milk Group: Two cups of milk equal two 8-ounce measuring cups. One cup low-fat plain yogurt may be substituted for 1 cup whole milk. One ounce hard or soft cheese may be substituted for 1 cup whole milk. One cup fat-free milk = 90 calories. One cup whole milk = 150 calories.

Fruits and Vegetables Group: One fruit serving equals 1 medium fruit, 2 small fruits, ½ banana, ¼ cantaloupe, 10–12 grapes or cherries, 1 cup fresh berries, or ½ cup fresh canned or frozen unsweetened fruit juice. Include one citrus fruit or other good source of vitamin C daily. One vegetable serving = ½ cup cooked or 1 cup raw leafy vegetable. Include one dark or deep yellow vegetable or other good source of vitamin A at least every other day. One fruit or vegetable serving = 50 to 75 calories.

Breads and Cereals Group: One serving equals 1 slice bread; 1 small dinner roll; ½ cup cooked cereal, noodles, macaroni, spaghetti, rice, or cornmeal; or 1 ounce (about ⅛ cup) ready-to-eat unsweetened fortified cereal. One bread or cereal serving = 75 calories.

Other: One serving equals 1 teaspoon butter, margarine, or oil; 6 nuts; or 2 teaspoons salad dressing. One serving = 35 to 50 calories.

Keep Your Muscles Strong

If you don't continue to exercise, your newly formed muscles will atrophy, or shrink, with disuse. Don't lose the muscle you worked so hard to gain.

Strong and shapely muscles are important to your midsection and throughout your body. Firm, toned muscles are your best insurance policy against regaining your lost fat.

The primary difference between muscle-maintenance and muscle-building routines is that you do not need workouts as frequently in maintenance mode. In other words, muscle is hard to build but easier to maintain.

To build muscle efficiently, you should exercise intensely twice a week. To maintain muscle, you only need to train once a week. You should still follow the negative-accentuated style with 15-15-15, plus 8 to 12 repetitions, that you've been doing for the last several months. You do not need to be as progressive in adding resistance or repetitions.

Keep in mind that more exercise is not necessarily better exercise. Better exercise is most often harder exercise. Apply this concept consistently and the tightness of your tummy may well exceed your goal.

Update and Evaluate Your Measurements

One final concept that you must follow up on is to keep accurate records of your ongoing measurements, especially your body weight and the three circumferences of your waist. Log and date these measurements in a notebook, so you can look back and evaluate your continued progression or stability.

You need to weigh yourself frequently, at least three times per week, usually first thing in the morning with nothing on. It's important to weigh yourself at roughly the same time every day because your weight fluctuates throughout the day. Expect some variation, perhaps from 1 to 3 pounds. This is normal. But any time you note an increase of 4 to 5 pounds, then it's time to double-check your calorie estimations and the specific foods you've consumed over the last several days.

You may be able to see what's happening better by taking weekly measurements of the three sites on your waist: 2 inches above the navel, at the navel, and 2 inches below the navel. Sometimes it's difficult to do these accurately by yourself, so you should probably get your workout partner and do these together. If one of those three waist measurements increases by 1 inch or more, it's time to start searching for some answers—and more importantly, move in a corrective direction. Reread Chapter 6 Nutrition for Fat Loss and get back on track.

The bottom line is that you've got to stay informed and motivated about maintenance, just like you were when you went through the program for the first time.

There is no easy path from fatness to fitness, not at the beginning, inter-mediate, advanced, or maintenance levels. Each one is challenging. But by following the principles of the Tighten Your Tummy program, you can achieve your fat-loss goals and maintain your wins for life. Read Roxanne's journal any time you need some inspiration to forge ahead.

chapter

18

Roxanne's Journal

My Journey to a Better Body

Roxanne Dybevick took top honors among the 41 women who participated in the Tighten Your Tummy 6-week program at Gainesville Health & Fitness, dropping a remarkable 23.27 pounds of fat. To help you better understand the experience, Roxanne shares selections from her journal.

Day 1: "Have a Strawberry, Just One?"

I'm not into weighing and measuring my body. And I had trouble believing that I weighed 164 pounds and had a waist that measured 36 inches. OMG! I absolutely need a smaller tummy.

I woke up early this morning excited to start the program. One thousand calories for a day is not something I have any concept of. The idea of being back to the size I was 20 pounds ago, before two children, is very appealing. The creator of the program is very inspiring. He has a lifetime of experience. That old idea that as I get older, I will get heavier and more out of shape doesn't have to be me. At least, that's my HOPE.

The detailed menu helped me find the food at the grocery store and see the plan coming alive. When I brought everything home, my family seemed to be eyeballing my food. I felt protective of my food. I could see I am going to need boundaries around my food. My household is busy: two teenagers, my husband, and my 81-year-old mother. It is a busy life here running to schools, my daughter's dance classes, and my son's community service commitment. My mother has had two heart attacks, a carotid endarterectomy, and 12 stents; she needs my help. On top of that, I have a diabetic, blind poodle, which needs two insulin shots 12 hours apart.

I am a stay-at-home mom/artist. Last weekend I was in a local fine art festival. Somehow I had 25 paintings in the show and sold all but three.

But I am committed to the Tighten Your Tummy program.

My 21st wedding anniversary is approaching, and I would like to be at the working-on-it stage, with some progress. I ate the approved first breakfast around 8:30 a.m. Now I have officially started. A toasted whole wheat bagel was surprisingly satisfying. I had eyeballed the correct amount of light cream cheese. Note: Get a food scale so I can actually measure the one ounce correctly.

I am allowed a cup of black coffee with this little meal. Now I must be honest, I normally end up at a Starbucks downing a cream-filled venti, so this is already very different behavior. The black coffee was surprisingly not too bad. I decided to eat at the table and try to make the best of it and enjoy the allotted food.

My husband comes along and sizes up my meal and says, "You should have a strawberry with that. It will make you in better shape for the day." Then he cocks his head and I know what my engineer means. He reasserts, "Have a strawberry, just one?"

I am trying to do the plan. He is trying to get me to eat a strawberry. I stand my ground, not really saying much at first, then after his insistence, I declare, "I am NOT eating a strawberry."

He lets it go. My first hurdle crossed.

Day 2: The Tighten Your Tummy Exercise Class

Today was the first group exercise class. I felt pretty good about it. We did the dreaded pushup-type exercise and also crunches and some sort of military plank body lowering slowly over this oversized coat hanger contraption, working the abs. I must admit, I have avoided the abdominal exercises at the gym. Fifteen years ago, I had a C-section and felt it was important to give the stitches time to really heal before starting abdominal crunches. I am thinking 15 years later, I'm probably good to go.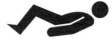

I've had two babies 2 years apart, so now I have two teenagers 2 years apart. Yes, you can say it: ugh. Trying to fit some ME time into my life is difficult.

Okay, I am whining. I will try and control that. Approaching the crunch bar thing was now a warrior woman who could move after all these years. I grabbed the handles on either side and thought, "How bad can this be? I could slip and sort of do a scooping move with my front teeth into the carpet or just sort of the major belly flop. Boom! Woman down, back row. Call the medics." It was really not so dramatic. I in a dignified manner turned my body into a solid plank while trying to listen to the directions the leader is giving us from the front of the room, while my arms are starting to tremble and bow out.

Time is called and I go from "Oh my" to I CAN DO THIS. I felt my heart pounding for a bit. It was amazing how some simple exercises can be so powerful. It also appears one side of my body wanted to cooperate with the directions more than the other side. So more of that on Wednesday.

Day 3: Plan Ahead for Success

Tuesday—I am off to visit a college campus with my son, so I find myself preparing the approved sandwich and afternoon snack to take with me. I am not sure when I will get back to town. I will also bring my handy-dandy cooler to keep my ice nearby for the water.

My mind starts overthinking the situation. If I am out longer than I plan, where am I going to find the approved dinner at a grocery store on the road? And then I will also need a microwave?

Second thought, bring the approved frozen microwave dinner with me, let it naturally thaw out during the day in the car. Then for the hours-long drive home, multitask, take a bungee cord, and strap the semi-thawed frozen approved dinner to the 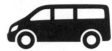 hood of my minivan and take the chill off that sucker. Pull over halfway home at a rest area, retrieve the meal, and eat my to-go dinner in the car. There is probably an unseen flaw in this plan. Note to self: Rethink the dinner plan.

What a busy day. I made it back home safely. It was a crazy day running around visiting the campus. I feel like I did pretty well staying on the plan. The water was easy. There seemed to be numerous opportunities to get ice and keep sipping. I left the campus later than I anticipated, starting the 2-hour drive home, realizing I would be waiting 2 hours to eat dinner to stay on the plan.

The water kept me from really getting that hungry. I just ate my approved snack and drank water all the way home.

Immediately, when I got home, I went straight to the freezer to get my dinner. I must admit it feels wonderful to eat when you are really hungry. I never realized that I have been eating without being hungry.

In fact, several times, while running around the various places on campus, I saw various snack foods and had the thought, I would be eating that if I was not on this plan.

This conscious thought made me realize how much snacking I was doing between meals. It has only been 3 days, but I have learned a lot about how I put on the extra pounds.

During my quick out-of-town day, I had several communications with team members, which helped keep me on track. This is a "we" plan. I need the support of my team. Thank you ladies!

Day 5: Bathroom Locator.com

Good morning. This is day 5 of the Tighten Your Tummy program. Drinking a gallon of ice water a day is proving to be a challenge. I am having images of myself in this tiny rowboat managing the rapids and white water crashing around me. Actually, it's me running to find a bathroom. Crashing through the door.

I am discovering which bathrooms around Gainesville I like best. We could share our personal favorites on a map, rating cleanliness, accessibility, and no waiting.

The beloved family poodle, Howie, is very confused by our changed relationship. In the past, we have had this cute little dance: I get my food, sit down at the table, and he comes over to be with me. He has this adorable begging routine that involves sitting back on his haunches, paws up, perfect attention. What a good boy. Actually rewarding begging at the table is probably not the best behavior to reward. But it is our thing.

Since I have been on the 1,000-calorie daily allowance, I find myself savoring every crumb. Each and every crumb is MINE. In fact, I have resorted to licking the plate. This is while our beloved, blind, diabetic, semi-bald, pancreatically challenged poodle is tilting his head to one side, giving me the most pathetic possible look that has ever existed.

I take the last bite and chew with passionate delight. Howie does not give up easily. After several minutes he starts wavering like a pine tree in the wind. This does not change his chances of receiving even a morsel.

Yes, it has come to this. Our relationship has changed. It is every man/dog for himself. In fact, I no longer see any need to cook for anyone. Note to self: Work on attitude—family is hungry.

Day 6: Coffee Is Kryptonite

I heard from one of the women in my group that the 1,000-calorie diet was going to get tougher. So I guess that day came a little earlier for me than expected. Yesterday was day 5. In the morning, after my nice approved bagel and finally getting my children to school, the moment of having a minute to actually think came.

You see thinking is the PROBLEM. The dreaded thought came, "I WANT COFFEE." And for me it is a deep hole. A free fall drenched in a splash of supercoated, white, luscious, cool, creamy half-and-half. No worries. Relax. I still have not broken my solemn vow. But I did drink a venti Starbucks BLACK cup of coffee yesterday. Very rugged.

This is my confession. Now I am free. How that Starbucks monster came to get my mind was like this—I overheard in the program exercise class Wednesday a woman asking if she could have HER "hot TEA in the morning." Personalizing it nicely.

She was asking about menu variations to the plan. The plan DOES NOT SAY TEA. She asked our fearless leader, Dr. Darden, with her head gently, in a sweet little sideways action to give further injection of a slightly pathetic tone and an "I need tea to live and stay on the plan" kind of look.

To my surprise, Dr. Darden said "YES" she could have tea, but no cream and sugar. I'm thinking, WIMP. My reptilian brain stored this little piece of information in a special place behind a locked door, in my MIND. Only special life situations freely open this padlocked door.

So I purchased a Starbucks coffee and brought the coffee back to my lair. Sat down to try and apply for an art show that has a 48-hour window left to sign up. I believe coffee is my Kryptonite.

From the URBAN Dictionary—Related to the *Superman* movies: Superman's weakness, it's the only thing that can hurt the man of steel. In other words, something you want but can't have can be called your Kryptonite.

Okay, got it. I have a very difficult time drinking coffee without EVIL HALF-AND-HALF.

Enough of that. I drank a cup of coffee, ALL RIGHT. Yes it was a big one. The written diet Dr. Darden gave us says we can have a cup of black coffee. I was exercising my right. This is when I know I have crossed the line: The rationalizing bad behavior starts, and the lying begins. I crossed the line.

Today is a new day. Note to self: Lighten up, be gentle on self. I did NOT eat the apple pie in the middle of the night my husband bought the second day of my diet. But yeah, I know. I got away with drinking the coffee BLACK but deeply, very deeply I wanted "MY CREAM." And I DO know that I did go to a slippery place.

Day 7: The Incredible Shrinking Woman

The morning has finally come, I am smaller. Laying in bed, I start to wake up and became vaguely aware that my tummy lump is not a beach ball anymore.

What happened? Did I do some sleepwalking, perhaps jogging program I am not aware of? In fact, my tummy seems more like I'm wearing a fanny pack—backwards.

BETTER. I look down under the sheets. Yes, the lump of fat is still there but seems to have changed shape. It seems lower and less. In fact, my entire abdominal area is not this bloated beach ball shape. I feel HOPE entering my soul.

Possibly I can control myself. This feeling of HOPE is new. I want it to expand and become me. Perhaps I have been covering up my true feeling for a very long time. After reviewing roving thoughts during the past week, I am realizing this fat problem is multi-layered. Literally.

This is what I have been wanting forever. THE ANSWER. THE TRUTH. The forest I have been lost in is filled with the past and the overwhelming responsibility of the present. In the middle of MY forest, I make decisions that take away my power. Shall I go left or right, do I eat it or not, or do I just sit here in the dark of the forest eating? Stuff down those emotions, stuff them down with ALL my might. Don't listen to my feelings as my clothes are getting tight. What am I feeding when I eat that cake?

The women in the program are talking about how much they weigh. And I do remember that one week ago, I weighed 164. And today, I feel and know I am lighter, much lighter. But it's just a number. As far as numbers, I am not a numbers kind of woman. In fact, I married the man who could balance my checkbook.

This is a task that is beyond my ability. Numbers are not my friends. In fact, I have probably weighed myself under 10 times in my life. It has never interested me. I seem to be VERY aware when I am heavier or thinner. I seem to have the clothes-fit-or-don't-fit method.

This seems to be an expensive method. It involves owning three sets of clothes. One set that is the size I would like to be,

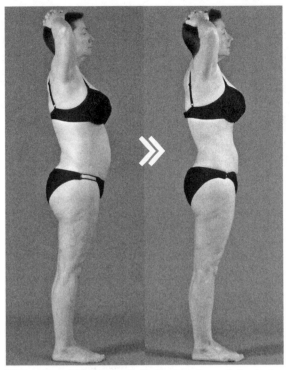

"Halfway through the program, Dr. Darden showed me my before-and-after photos, which were taken at the end of 2 weeks. I was amazed. My after stomach looked so much smaller, tighter, and better."

the next size is the size I sort of am. And the next is the size I wear when I want to be absolutely comfortable.

Today I feel FREE, with endless possibilities. I am going to go paint. I have set up three art shows to keep busy as I slide into my new size. I want to stay busy. Interestingly enough, I am having the desire to paint food. I'm going with this. First it will be a doughnut with pink frosting on a pretty white plate. God help me. LOL. Ladies, keep me close.

Day 9: Irrational Thought

The week is getting off to a calm start, comforting. Living with two teenagers, I look for these calm moments. Probably instead of enjoying them, I am partially wondering when the other shoe will drop. I have had the irrational thought: What if I completely follow the diet and the exercises and I don't lose any weight. Yes, this is not thinking clearly.

But the thought has crossed my mind. What if I have the kind of fat that is like waterproof plastic—no amount of ice water, exercise, hard work, sacrifice, following the rules will budge it. I went to the Internet and looked up general information about a 1,000-calorie diet, and it seemed reassuring that this regimen would produce results.

We were weighed and measured the first day of the program and photographed. That is a documented moment in history. On Sunday, October 12, 2014, 9:45 am, a photo exists of exactly what I look like.

The raw truth—stomach rolling, breasts toppling, arms flapping, here I am world. I was so excited to be doing something about the problem, I didn't actually find out what I weighed or what my body fat was. I was weighed and measured but have no idea. This seems to be a pattern in my life. Note to self: Pay attention!

Probably just getting into a bikini after 20 years was enough reason to forget any details like, how much do I actually weigh. I know Dr. Darden has the information. I remember standing there in this little black string bikini bottom and a borrowed top. My stomach felt like it was walking in front of me and I was somewhere behind one or two steps, and my breasts were these enormous footballs I have been trying to control. They were toppling over the edge of the bikini top, straining to stay under wraps.

One thing I will love about being thinner will be having smaller breasts. I have no understanding of what all the breast fascination in the world is about. I have spent a lifetime carrying around more than I want. Admiring small breasts all my life. In fact, when painting, I always paint the breasts I would like to have. A nice perky A-B cup. As I have gained weight, I have gone from a B, maybe C to a DD. This difference is not welcome.

Over the weekend looking for entertainment, I borrowed my mother's digital scale. She bought the scale after her second heart attack.

I have learned a lot about heart disease in the last 10 years. From my mother, 81, and my husband's grandmother, 97. The scale is in mint condition. I don't believe she has ever stepped on it. My mother has different problems. She is struggling to stay above 105 pounds. Her two food groups are coffee and chocolate. This is for another entry. I will say learning healthy eating habits is not what I learned from her.

Okay, enough guilt sloshing. I am taking responsibility today for my life, my weight, and my future. Stepping out into the clearing, my past family patterns need not sabotage me. The self-talk today is, I CAN DO THIS, I HAVE VALUE, I HAVE EVERYTHING I NEED, I CAN CONTROL MYSELF.

Note to self: The best years of my life lie ahead. There are no accidents. I am exactly where I need to be.

Day 10: Lucky 7

Today is day 10 of the tighter tummy program. Yesterday we had our regular 30-minute Monday exercise class. Entering the gym, I go to the locker room and weigh myself. Deciding every ounce counts, I strip down to underwear and bra to get a more accurate number. The starting number was 164 pounds, and then using my mother's borrowed scale, I was ready to get the true number.

Nine days on the 1,000-calorie diet produced new and exciting results. Some quick math and I realize I have lost 7 pounds. A layer of self-doubt falls away. I have HOPE. This is really exciting. This was not LUCK, wishful thinking, prayer, surgery, or my imagination. I have lost 7 pounds. Yes, this is the beginning, but I really needed some good news.

The difference between my husband and me is enormous. Last March, I started commenting to my husband he was starting to look pregnant. I had never really seen him carry extra fat. We have been together a long time, and he always seems to be in control of his mouth. Not just his mouth, but frankly in control of himself.

But this past year, he had put on a few pounds and had taken a different shape. I'm thinking, okay, he's getting fatter, I'm getting fatter. Looks like we will be old butterballs together. But I must admit, I was slightly enjoying joking about his belly. For once he was not perfect. I had a foothold.

Until sometime after March, I crossed the line and had an

overhang belly that surpassed his belly. Then it wasn't funny anymore. The year is going by and it is May or June, and I look at my husband and I realize he looks different. He has lost weight. Silently he started his own program. Hitting the gym, changing his eating habits. I believe this is called SELF-CONTROL. This is not something that I have a lot of experience with.

He has dropped 20 pounds. I ask him, "How the HELL did you do that?" He very quietly, calmly, scientifically, and deliberately described his plan of action. Daily he did a 300–400 calorie workout and reduced his calorie intake 200–300 calories.

I'm like, that is not fair. He never joined a group, he never asked for support, never moaned about the difficulties he faced keeping his act together while holding his complicated professional career, our family, and his act together while he dropped the weight. This is Norwegian, I suspect.

This is not me. I need to have an entire room of people who are going through the same thing I am going through. I need to talk about what is on my mind. It is my mind that is against me. Left alone with my thoughts, I can rationalize unhealthy behavior.

Yes, tell myself RATIONAL LIES. So, I need my bright orange tank top that my little weight loss program team created. The one that says CRUNCH BUNCH. It makes me feel part of the inside track. The one that makes me feel part of the solution. Thank you, team.

Day 11: 21 Years

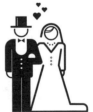

Yesterday was my 21st anniversary. Yes, 21 years ago I got married. For the third time. That doesn't sound good. I could say, "The first two don't count" and then that sounds even worse.

Yesterday afternoon I was realizing my husband would come home, and we need to do some type of celebration for getting to 21 years. Since a big sweet cake is off the table—and any other sweet treat—it is like, what do we do with ourselves? He TEXTS me toward the end of the afternoon, "WE CAN WALK TO THE GYM AND EAT LIGHT TO CELEBRATE."

This is what it has come to. It is really just another day. Relax, I tell myself. The cruise, the sun-splashed surprise weekend, the fun dinner out, alone—no kids—up in smoke.

Our life is a series of smaller decisions that can, in my mind, place me in a position to be hurt or not. It is my decision. In fact, I ate the unnecessary calories that made me overweight to begin with, that made me fatter than I want to be, that eventually enrolled me in the tighter tummy 1,000-calorie diet plan, on my anniversary. Once again, here we are.

Practice letting go. Let go of all my ideas about what I think would satisfy me? There it is, the problem. How do I satisfy myself? Is it painting a masterpiece, having a passion-filled weekend away from responsibility, having my sister take care of OUR mother for a few months?

Still, I think losing 20 pounds trumps everything. And thanks to Dr. Darden, I am working on that. In fact, today, I put on pants that felt roomy. What a beautiful feeling. To button the button.

Day 13: Body-Mind Makeover

One step in front of the other, here we go. At the beginning of the year, I decided, this is the year I am going to get it together. After several ill-fated get-it-together plans, I am at the end of October and finally making progress. To be honest, my progress has all taken place in the last 13 days.

This week has been all about staying on the diet and trying to complete this painting. At my last art show, I took an unfinished painting to work on while sitting at my booth. I managed to sell it unfinished. So now I am trying complete it. Frankly my concentration has not been that good. It seems like my mind has been kind of racing, thinking, thinking, thinking. I contacted the buyer, and she is picking up the painting this weekend. Thank God.

It seems like grazing on snacks, obtaining snacks, and thinking about what I will snack on was occupying a great deal of time. In fact, I am pretty sure it was some sort of self-soothing behavior. There is a new rawness to life that comes from halting this feeding frenzy. As I am getting smaller my ideas are getting bigger. I purchased an enormous canvas. Not entirely sure what I am going to paint, but it is going to be BIG.

Growing up, my mother had absolutely NO sweets in our house. The only time we ever had anything sweet was holidays. But the rest of the year, we didn't have candy, cookies, chips, soda, or any sweets. Looking back on this, I asked my mom about her mothering decisions regarding what food to have in the house. My son always seemed to be a picky eater. So I asked Mom, "How did you get my sister and I so willing to eat just about anything?" Mom described her growing up and how food was handled.

Well, it turns out my mother was hospitalized for not eating in her youth. This was news to me. My grandmother and grandfather were VERY strict. You had to eat everything on your plate, and if you didn't, the same plate was brought out again, at the next meal, for you to THEN FINISH THE MEAL.

This routine went on and on. Many times, they would bring the same plate out, night after night, until it was eaten. Also she described being tied to the chair so she would not be able to leave the table. I look at my mom and say, "WHAT? You have got to be kidding?"

Until I became a mother myself, and started trying to feed people, and my mother and I had that conversation, I had no idea what a problem food was for her. In fact, she managed to hide it from me my entire life, that she does not eat anything green.

About 10 years ago, she sold her house and built on to my house. So we have ALL been living together for a while. Mom told me that she didn't really know what to feed my sister and me growing up, but she knew she didn't want to do to us what was done to her. She thought if she eliminated sweets from the equation, she would be better able to eventually figure out what to feed us. My mom was a single mom in the '60s navigating, trying to work, and raising two children alone. My dad died when I was one year old.

I love knowing what I am going to eat each day. I really didn't know it was such a burden. But then I still have the what-is-everyone-else-going-to-eat problem. My daughter is vegetarian, my husband is semi-vegetarian, my son a carnivore, and, as I said before, my mother seems to be surviving on chocolate and coffee—sprinkled with a few meals I try to bring her that she hides in her microwave.

Anyway, food is complicated around here. I do feel like creating meals is an enormous challenge. Sometimes I am really trying, and then sometimes I have had enough trying to figure out what everyone will eat. I am close to "every man for himself."

Note to self: Try and work on a new attitude about cooking for family.

Day 14: Navigating the MIND Field

It is Saturday evening and I am home safe. Last night, I survived a sticky chocolate covered Art Reception, where BIG bowls of individually wrapped mini-size chocolate bars loomed and later, a CHIC-BURGER joint, WITH EVERY TOPPING IMAGINABLE. TODAY, a cheese-covered pizzeria.

In fact, I can still see the cute couple sitting next to us, in love, beautiful, their lives ahead of them, a 20-something super slim woman, trying to navigate her first slice out of the pie. She takes her piece, trying to control the long, golden cheese string. Arching her back, laughing, ha, ha, ha, it is so funny, she successfully stuffs the cheese string into her perfect lips, licking her long lean polished nails, together they shrug their shoulders, how funny.

I'm having an out-of-body experience. Okay, that's it, I have had enough, I'm watching PIZZA PORN. I get a text from a woman in the program, "Keep up the good work." I excuse myself from my family and walk outside the restaurant for a breath of fresh, non-pizza-filled air. My family is eating a 3:00 p.m. meal, and it's not on my plan.

This morning I put on a pair of jeans and realized the jeans didn't fit. Could it be true? I start searching for the next size down. Yes, the glorious moment has arrived. This pair of jeans I left behind a while ago is now fitting again. They feel like an old friend.

For a very long time, the search has gone the other way. Trying to get dressed, putting on several outfits, and deciding I look too fat. This morning I realized I am going in the right direction. I am going to make a pile of clothes to go to Goodwill.

You will hear from me weekly, each Sunday, from now on. Until the end of our program. I'll be focusing on painting and doing the Tighten Your Tummy program together. Thank you for staying with me. I'm looking forward to a thrilling conclusion. What a gift, to be excited about my life.

Day 22: The Coyote in the Attic

It might seem like a strange title for an entry in my diary, but it makes perfect sense to me. In fact, I think the Coyote in the Attic pretty much sums it up. Sort of like the ELEPHANT in the LIVING ROOM.

After addressing my demons directly for the past 22 days, I am more clearly seeing the family patterns that have dictated my thinking behaviors that have in turn contributed to the layer of fat residing on my body. My mother grew up during the era of the "CLEAN PLATE CLUB." President Herbert Hoover knew that many Americans had a strong sense of patriotism during the war, trying to protect scarce food supplies and use supplies more efficiently. He used this to his advantage when he advertised the idea of the "Clean Plate" campaign.

In a previous entry, I described how my mother was actually physically restrained, tied to the chair at the table, and asked to eat her meal. If not eaten completely, then that plate was brought out night after night until it was eaten, every single morsel. My mother's treatment was an act of patriotism and a way her parents contributed to the success of the United States.

All this in a plate of food. I believe we are ALL members of the club, whether we know it or not.

Recently, my mother and I were driving around town running errands, and I casually asked her what INTERESTING things happened to her at the dinner table growing up. I was expecting some stimulating historical family dinner conversation that might have happened around my grandparents' table. What my mother described was QUITE interesting.

Mother described during the Depression when people were out of jobs, they would come by the house and ask for work—to try and earn money for FOOD. This was a frequent occurrence. My mother's family was living in Lafayette, Indiana, in a large historic-type home. The type of home that could house a family of four plus room for hired help.

My mother then mentions a woman coming by the house and needing a place to live and my grandmother, having a big heart, agreeing she could live in the attic and work around the house for her keep. This woman then asked if her pet could come along and explained that it would be no trouble. Her pet turned out to be a coyote.

My mother goes on to detail the family sitting around the table eating a meal. The whole family attended grandma's dinners, with all the formality involved in being an army officer's wife. Grandpa at one end of the table and Grandma at the other end. The family circled around. The coyote living in the attic, baying, as the crystal water glasses on the table are vibrating to the soulful, mournful, wailing sound.

I believe the coyote in the attic was actually trying to communicate with other coyotes. Except we were living in the city, and there were no other coyotes in the area. So what they had in the attic was a lonely, frustrated coyote. This went on for some time, and the family went on with their business of living, and conversations were elevated to hear each other above the nonstop soulful howl.

The coyote, however, might have been asking other coyotes to come and help my mother. To take her away to the safety of the coyote den where she could eat when hungry and express herself freely. Had the coyote been successful in contacting his pack, perhaps this story would have had a different ending.

Anyway, the point is today, families are still members of the "Clean Plate Club." I believe it is time to disband the club. My mother, at 81 years old, still looks for the smallest plate in the house to eat on, as if the old club rules are still in effect.

Today is the halfway point in the program, and I must admit, in just 3 short weeks, my attitude has completely changed. I find myself empowered as a woman, feeling like I

AM BACK. Yes BACK in the game. The layer of fat was smothering my confidence and crushing my dreams. I had become literally someone I didn't recognize. I have lost 15 pounds. I have not cheated ONCE on the program, and I am pleased by the results.

The BIGGEST change has not been my weight but my feelings about myself. I have adapted to the new way of living. The PROGRAM. It is a commitment. A commitment to myself. To my health. And to my future.

Day 29: The Romance Is OVER

How quickly I can forget the life I led just a month ago. The scrounging around trying to find something to wear that concealed the truth has ended. As the old ME disappears and the new ME emerges, a confidence has come over me. I have regained my footing. I am becoming aware of the strong need I have for rewarding myself with food. Learning to love myself at each stage of the transformation.

Our society views food as LOVE. Food is considered an important way to show affection. The real question becomes how to love myself without overeating. How to disconnect the message center in my brain that tells me I have to eat with others to excess, to feel the love.

I have been in many slippery, fat-filled events over the past month and not broken my solemn vow. Last night while attending my sister's birthday party, I brought my approved meal, popped it in her microwave, and was thinking how great it felt to have control of myself.

I sat and watched my mother, who is a heart patient, eat breaded sweet and sour pork, lemon tart, raspberry tart, and ice cream. That would have been me, if it were not for my determination. There was much discussion about the food, the pre-meal food talk, oohing and awing, then the shuffling of plates, then the loading of the food.

I heated my meal in silence. Reserving any comment. I am on a mission. After my breakup with Reese's Peanut Butter Cups at

Halloween 2 weeks ago, I am strengthened knowing I didn't eat even ONE out of an enormous bowl for trick-or-treaters.

As a serious contender in the Tighten Your Tummy program's overall Top Loser, I have had to forgo these bonding sessions. And chew my meal slowly and make it last, getting every amount of pleasure I can possibly extract from a turkey sandwich. And when the sandwich is gone, it is gone. I am NOT consuming the crunchy meal-extending chips.

There were several people at the birthday party that had not seen me since I started the tighter tummy program. One person mentioned that I looked REALLY GOOD, eyeing me up and down, trying to figure out what had changed. For one, my face seems to have slimmed down considerably. They are seeing the weight change, but more significantly, they are encountering a new me.

Over and over as I run into friends, who are giving me this second look, I find myself looking people straight in the eye. Wanting an authentic communication. I am coming out of hiding. Whatever I am protecting doesn't need protecting any longer. What I am is good enough. I am enough. What I am experiencing is a relationship with myself because the romance with food is OVER.

Day 36: Less Is More

I weigh less, yet I feel like more. More excited about life. More in control. More attractive. More healthy. More in charge. More successful. Basically, MORE ME. Imagine that. In every positive way, I am MORE, just by the simple undeniable fact there is LESS of ME.

In fact, being fat was a HUGE problem for me. It took every ounce of denial to convince myself everything was FINE. It was the last 2 years where I had crossed the line. I went from a little over to plump. Yes I said the "P" word.

In the last 5 weeks, I have learned I am capable of being satisfied with less. Imagine that. Less calories. Eat less and listen less to the self-sabotaging voice within. To be successful on the Dr. Darden plan, I have had to go inside and perform some emotional surgery.

Friday night was a formal business dinner for my husband's work. Spouses were invited for everyone to get to know each other. I knew in advance this was an occasion I wanted to look really together for: slim, successful, and comfortable. Last year I attended a similar event with him, remembering I was not very happy about the outfit I wore. Spending most of the night sucking in my gut so hard it was hard to relax. Somehow during last year's event, I was able to rearrange the reality in my mind and carry on the mindless eating and follow with cheesecake for full caloric intake. When I can't breathe from the pressure on my gut, give me the cheesecake.

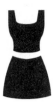

The dinner party was an interesting experience in self-control. I was unable to bring my frozen approved meal, so I had to do the math. It was actually pretty easy. During the social time at the bar area, I sipped Perrier. Safe there. Then, for the sit-down dinner part, I ate three scallops, no cream sauce, and rice. I think the portion was very similar to our evening approved meal.

Then, a person sitting next to us at the table strikes up a conversation with me. "So what is it that you do?"

I'm thinking, quickly—think of what I do. Clearing my throat I say, "I am a stay-at-home mother/artist." What I am thinking is, "I have been overeating at home for a while, gotten fat, and have been on Dr. Darden's diet program for 5 weeks, lost 17 pounds, and think I look pretty good tonight. What do you think?" Okay, he probably doesn't want to hear all about it.

The plates are cleared, and the dessert portion of the formal dinner starts. Now what do I do, sitting next to my husband, who has lost 35 pounds on the hard-core Norwegian weight-loss program designed by himself? By the way, I don't recommend his plan. Then, he says, "My wife and I will take our desserts home in a box please." I'm like, well, that was pretty smart. I wouldn't have thought of that.

We are off the hook, except we get to watch everyone else lick and prod their ooey gooey, crème brûlée with drizzled caramel. WHATEVER. I am over it. It felt absolutely wonderful to love what I was wearing and feel comfortable.

The program has given me a genuine gratitude for the food I have been eating. I approach my approved meals in a new and appreciative way. I take very small bites and chew slowly, enjoying each bite. Not rushing at all. I am capable of extending my meal quite a bit. By taking the time to slow down and focus. This new practice leaves me quite satisfied with the new meal portion size. No rushing, face stuffing, to-go meal action going on. I am taking the time to nourish my body, enjoy my meal.

This practice is one decision in a series of small decisions. Remembering to practice the self-care—it is ALL a series of small decisions, each day, as I make clear choices to practice loving myself. And stand firmly in the clearing.

Day 43: Yes, I Made a Decision

Today was our after weigh-in on the program. I arrived at the fitness center for the final photo session with an enormous sense of accomplishment. I dropped 17.3 pounds of body weight. Plus, I had a muscle gain of 5.97 pounds, which according to Dr. Darden's calculations means I actually lost 23.27 pounds of fat.

I remember from my drawing classes that an adult human head weighs 8 pounds, and I've lost three heads of solid fat. I am astonished by that visual.

Six weeks ago, when I heard about the Tighten Your Tummy program, I thought, "This is exactly what I need." What a giant understatement.

This was the beginning of me realizing it's time to address my tummy. I knew after the C-section, they said I should wait 6 weeks to do any exercising so I don't hurt myself. Well I waited 15 years. Since starting the inner-ab vacuum exercises before eating major meals and the abdominal crunches, my abs have emerged and come alive. I know I still have work to do, but after losing 23 pounds, I can see what the next steps are. When I sit down, the rolls of fat are gone. This is very motivating. Empowering.

I must say I will miss the friends I have made in the weekly exercise classes. We went through something together. Something much bigger than merely losing the weight. We all had suffered the emotional and physical pain of being overweight. And together we all recovered a part of ourselves that had been covered over.

I am continuing on and will now take this to the next level. Christmas is in about a month, and I have a beautiful start to having a nice set of abs for Christmas.

Now that the layer of fat is gone, I am totally motivated to continue to strengthen the foundation I have started. Thank you Dr. Darden. This Tighten Your Tummy program has been life changing. I am forever grateful. And it is my decision to take a stand daily and take care of myself and continue practicing what you have taught me.

Yes, I made a decision, and it changed my life.

chapter
19

All Your Questions Answered

Specifics to Help You Succeed

Following are some of the frequently asked questions raised by test panel participants and others about the Tighten Your Tummy program. If you don't find your answers here, post your question to me at DrDarden.com. I'll put my best science and experience into each response.

Down-Up-Down Calories

Q: Your 2-week Power-Start Diet limits calories to 1,000 a day. Then it increases to 1,200 calories for 2 weeks and drops to 1,100 calories a day for the final 2 weeks. Why not just keep the entire 6 weeks at an average 1,100 calories a day? Wouldn't that be simpler?

A: You're right. That would simplify the eating plan. But here's my reasoning:

Starting with just 1,000 calories for the first 2 weeks takes resolve and discipline, which is often strongest at the start of a program. And even more importantly, it reinforces my concept that inactivity on a reduced-calorie diet is necessary for efficient fat loss. You cannot be very active on just 1,000 calories a day. More rest is part of the answer to being successful during Weeks 1 and 2.

Then, during Weeks 3 and 4, the extra 200 calories a day provides an "energy surge" to the average female dieter and offers a psychological lift that spurs additional motivation. I've found that asking dieters to reduce by 100 calories a day for Weeks 5 and 6 helps them refocus their discipline and dedication for a final push.

In summary, the down-up-down plan offers more variety, intellectual stimulation, and overall excitement than a straight 1,100 calories a day for 42 consecutive days. Over the last 40 years, I've tried both methods on groups of women, and I believe the 1,000-1,200-1,100 plan, or down-up-down variations of it, works best.

Vegetarian Guidelines

Q: Can a vegetarian follow the Tighten Your Tummy eating plan?

A: Of course! Remember, unlike a lot of currently popular high-protein diets, this one emphasizes more high-quality carbohydrates. So a vegetarian can do very well on Tighten Your

Tummy. In fact, two of my test panelists, Brianna Kramer and Sara Smith, are vegetarians. Both know a lot about food and nutrition and how to make the necessary adjustments.

The key is to be sure you're getting enough of the other macronutrients, protein and fat, when eating a vegetarian diet. You can do that by eating legumes like black, red, pinto, and other beans; nut butters; and nuts. Make stir-fry meals with tofu. Create delicious sandwiches using hummus made from chickpeas. To make dinners fast and easy and take advantage of automatic portion control, choose frozen microwaveable dinners. You'll find many good vegetarian offerings by browsing Michelinas.com, Leancuisine.com, and Healthychoice.com.

Physical Attraction

Q: Your early chapters suggest that improving one's physical attractiveness is the main goal of tightening your tummy. Is that true? It bothers me that so much emphasis is placed on appearance in our society.

A: I agree that we are a society that often values looks and style above substance. That may be unfortunate, but it's reality. The *Glamour* magazine article "How Do You Feel About Your Body?" which I discussed in Chapter 2, clearly shows that more women today are unhappy with their body than a similar group surveyed in 1984.

Most women diet and exercise because they want to improve their shape and make themselves more attractive. I think that is a fine motivation for getting in shape, but increased physical attractiveness is only one of the benefits of strength-training exercise and having a smaller tummy. As I mentioned earlier in the book, a flat belly has been an outward sign of health and fertility for thousands of years. And the health benefits of losing belly fat are well established. A woman who eats and trains properly can also expect to:

- Increase her muscular strength

- Enhance her flexibility

- Improve the function of her heart and lungs

- Develop better posture

- Become more proficient in almost any sport

- Augment her energy

- Recuperate faster than average from illness or injury

- Look and feel better by shaping her muscles to their maximum potential

- Build a more positive self-image

- Reduce anxiety and combat depression

- Avoid or even reverse prediabetes and diabetes

Whatever your goals are—improving your looks or your health (or both!)—negative-accentuated exercise will help you achieve them in the most efficient manner.

"I'm fairly attractive," wrote another woman, "and at times become disgusted with men who tell me, 'You're very attractive, and I'd like to know you better.' Whatever happened to intelligence and charm?"

Intelligence and charm are still desirable. But according to Ellen Berscheid, PhD, a professor of psychology at the University of Minnesota who has studied the effects of physical attractiveness for more than 40 years, intelligence and charm have definitely taken a backseat to physical beauty.

In other words, do not underestimate the importance of how you look.

Dr. Berscheid concludes that the importance of physical attractiveness will continue to grow as increases in geographical mobility, frequent job changes, and divorce subject more people to one-time or few-time interactions with others. Just as most people judge a book by its cover, they also form lasting opinions of others from appearance alone.

Most people have little control over the social behavior of others. But you can try to understand the reasoning behind some of the behavior, whether you agree with it or not, and intelligently work with it to reach your goals.

Determining Waist-to-Hip Ratio

Q: About the waist-to-hip ratio of 0.7: Exactly how is that determined?

A: Your waist-to-hip ratio is fairly easy to determine. With an ordinary cloth or plastic tape, measure the circumference of your waist (in inches and eighths of an inch) at the smallest level, which is usually in the neighborhood of 2 inches above your navel. Stand tall and don't suck in your waist during the measurement. Then, while standing with your feet together, measure the circumference of your hips at the maximum protrusion level. Write both of those measurements down on a sheet of paper.

Divide the waist measurement by the hip measurement, which will provide you with a ratio. For example, your waist may measure 34.25 inches and your hips may measure 41 inches. So 34.25 divided by 41 equals 0.835, which rounds off to 0.84. If you look at yourself in a full-length mirror, it's the on-the-side curve—indicated by that 0.7 ratio—that Devendra Singh found was so important in a female's sexual attractiveness.

Let's look at some different ratios, which were roughly generated from my test panel's averages, with the hip measurement remaining the same:

41/41 = 1.0	35/41 = 0.85
39/41 = 0.95	33/41 = 0.8
37/41 = 0.9	**31/41 = 0.76**

$$29/41 = 0.71 \qquad\qquad 25/41 = 0.61$$

$$27/41 = 0.66 \qquad\qquad 24/41 = 0.59$$

Singh noted that as the waist-to-hip ratio got smaller, at least up to a point, the on-the-side curve increased and the female improved her attractiveness. The bolded measurements—with the ratios of 0.76, 0.71, and 0.66—were in the almost-ideal range, with 0.7 being ideal.

Singh would no doubt be interested in the extreme attention that Kim Kardashian generates with measurements of approximately 25/43, which would equal the low ratio of 0.58. Plus, two more celebrities, Nicki Minaj and Coco Austin, have published measurements of 26/45 and 23/40, which would equal ratios of 0.57 and 0.57.

These low ratios are certainly classified as extreme hourglass shapes, which differ significantly from the classic movie stars of yesterday—such as Lana Turner, Marilyn Monroe, and Brigitte Bardot—each with their ideal 0.7 ratios and measurements of 24/34.5, 26/37, and 24.5/35 (author's estimates).

Also, remember that my daughter, Sarah, whose measurements were noted on page 2, was the only woman in the group of 41 with a waist that measured 24 inches. Her waist-to-hip ratio was 0.67, with measurements of 24.5/36.75.

More on Carbohydrates

Why Carbs Are Key

Q: **I'm confused. All of my girlfriends avoid eating carbohydrates to lose weight. Please help me understand why carbohydrates are essential in fat loss?**

A: I appreciate where you are coming from and I know how tough it is to go against what many of your friends believe and practice. Normally, a complete discussion of the importance of carbohydrates in a college nutrition textbook would take 20 pages or more. I'm going to condense it to five paragraphs and hope that you get the essence of why carbs are key. Let's begin by examining glucose.

Glucose: Glucose is the basic carbohydrate unit used for energy by each of your body's cells. The cells of your brain and nervous system depend almost exclusively on glucose, and your red blood cells use glucose alone. What you need to know is that only dietary carbohydrates release glucose and that's why carbs are classified as an *essential nutrient*. For vigorous health, you need plenty of them each day to power your body and brain.

Lack of carbohydrates: Although you can eat too many carbohydrates and the extra glucose can be converted to body fat, body fat cannot be converted to glucose to feed your brain adequately. When your body faces a severe carbohydrate deficit, it has two problems. Having no glucose, it has to make glucose from proteins—which, because of proteins' critical functions, it does not like to do, even in emergencies. When it is forced to do so, it pulls proteins from your organs and muscles—which makes no sense, especially if you are interested in fitness and health. Carbohydrates should be available to prevent your body stealing proteins from your muscles for energy. This is called the *protein-sparing action* of carbohydrates. Remember, protein builds muscles and muscle burns a lot of calories. If your body cannibalizes its muscle to make glucose to feed your brain, you compromise one of your body's prime natural calorie burners. You need adequate carbohydrates every day. Don't starve yourself of carbs but do choose them wisely.

Ketone bodies: The second problem with a lack of dietary carbohydrates is a precarious shift in your body's energy metabolism. Instead of following the carbohydrate-energy pathway, fats are forced to fragment and combine with each other—which causes an accumulation of normally scarce acidic products called ketone bodies. Ketone bodies can accumulate in the blood to disturb the normal acid-base balance, which then may promote deficiencies of vitamins and minerals, elevate blood cholesterol, and yield little energy. As a result, most low-carbohydrate dieters soon feel lethargic and have poor motivation.

Minimum recommendation for carbohydrates: To provide glucose, preserve proteins (and muscle mass), and avoid ketone bodies, you need to consume adequate carbohydrates each day. According to scientists at the DRI (Dietary Reference Intakes for healthy women in the United States and Canada), the minimum amount of dietary carbohydrates is 130 grams—which equals 520 calories of carbohydrate-rich foods each day. The Tighten Your Tummy menus furnish 520 calories or more each day of carbohydrate-rich foods—such as fruits, vegetables, and whole grains.

In summary, for effective fat loss and efficient tummy tightening, a healthy woman needs at least 130 grams of carbohydrates a day to do the following: Supply glucose for brain alertness, initiate protein-sparing action, prevent ketone bodies, and provide energy for training and daily activities. The Tighten Your Tummy diet contains the right amount of carbohydrates, combined with proteins, fats, and water to make your journey successful.

Q: **Are you saying all of the popular low-carbohydrate diets do not work?**

A: What I'm saying is these diets, without adequate carbohydrates, do not work competently in losing fat. If you are only interested in losing weight, not fat, then eliminating carbohydrates will result in a loss of water from your body. Remember, carbohydrates are *hydrated* carbons. Each ounce of glucose carries with it 3 ounces of water. Go on a low-carbohydrate diet for a week and you may lose 5 or 6 pounds of water weight. The water, however, will not drain from your fat. It will come from you organs and muscles. But the typical low-carbohydrate dieter won't recognize that detail.

Since most overfat women rarely endure strict low-carbohydrate dieting on their own for longer than 2 weeks, the initial scale drop from the loss of water provides them with a false sense of achievement. Many then believe that if they had continued longer, they would have reached their goal. Thus, their low-carbohydrate eating practices appear to work when in fact they don't, and these beliefs continue to be reinforced.

As I discussed in Chapters 2 and 3, your goal should be to lose fat and build your underlying muscles. In fact, building muscle at the same time as you are losing weight assures that your weight loss comes from your fat cells. That's one of the primary reasons a carbohydrate-rich eating plan is important in tummy tightening.

Eating plans that advise people to avoid carbohydrates supplied by fruits, vegetables, and breads should be ignored. Enjoying tasty carbohydrates within your calorie limit each day is a part of the Tighten Your Tummy diet. As you progress through the complete program—and see and feel significant results—you'll appreciate carbohydrates more and more.

The Science of Getting Stronger

Q: **What causes a muscle to become stronger?**

A: There are three basic types of muscles. The skeletal muscles are used for body movement and are under voluntary, conscious control. The heart, automatically operated by the nervous system and not under conscious control, is composed of another kind of tissue called cardiac muscle. A third type, called smooth muscle, automatically serves internal functions, propelling food through the stomach and constricting blood vessels to adjust blood flow. The three types of muscles are interrelated, but only the voluntary skeletal muscles benefit directly from exercise. Cardiac muscle is strengthened by proper exercise, but the effect is secondary, as a result of increased demand on the circulatory system by the skeletal muscles. Skeletal muscles, therefore, are the key to overall body shape and fitness.

The skeletal muscles are composed of millions of strands of a thin filament protein called actin and a thick filament protein called myosin. Given the presence of calcium, magnesium, and two other proteins called troponin and tropomyo-

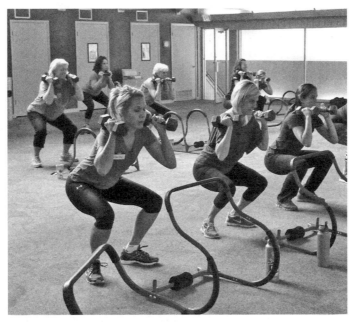

The dumbbell squat, performed in the 15-15-15 style, targets the strongest muscles in the entire body: the gluteals, hamstrings, and quadriceps. These muscles should always be worked intensely—even if your focus is primarily on your abdominal region.

sin, actin and myosin can contract and move your limbs with great force.

The fuel for muscular contraction is a chemical compound called adenosine triphosphate, or ATP. When one of the three phosphates has broken off from ATP to form ADP, or adenosine diphosphate, energy is released into the muscular environment. When the actin binds to myosin in the presence of calcium, the energy released from ATP breakdown is used to pull the actin filaments along the myosin filaments. More specifically, a bridge forms between actin and myosin. Energy from ATP breakdown is used to shorten the actomyosin cross-bridge, which shortens the muscle.

When muscle is contracted repeatedly against resistance, it overcompensates by growing larger and stronger. The technical term for muscular growth is hypertrophy. The signal for hypertrophy is intensity of contraction, and the negative phase of the exercise is clearly the best way to intensify the process.

When a muscle is faced with high-intensity requirements, it responds with a protective increase in muscular size and strength.

When hypertrophy happens, a number of physical changes occur that cause increased muscular size and strength:

- The actin and particularly the myosin protein filaments increase in size.

- The number of actin/myosin units increases.

- The number of blood capillaries within the fiber may increase.

- The amount of connective tissue may increase.

This is rather complicated, but in short, when individual muscle fibers increase their volume by adding actin and myosin, the muscle grows larger and stronger. The total number of muscle fibers, however, remains the same.

Gluten Sensitive

Q: **I'm sensitive to gluten. Is there any way I can adapt your diet for me?**

A: Yes. There are two Web sites I'll list later that can help you adapt my Tighten Your Tummy diet. But first you need to be aware of the following.

Consumer Reports published a five-page article, "Will a Gluten-Free Diet Really Make You Healthier?" which points out that only about 7 percent of Americans can't eat gluten because they have celiac disease or a diagnosed gluten sensitivity. This is in contrast to a third of Americans who say they buy and consume gluten-free foods.

The article says that for most people living in the United States, a gluten-free diet can pose risks. Researchers reviewed nutrition labels for more than 80 gluten-free foods. A few of the concerns: Some gluten-free foods contain more fat, sugar, or sodium than their regular counterparts.

For example, *Consumer Reports* tested a gluten-free bagel with 7 grams of fat. A regular bagel had just 2 grams. While products made of enriched wheat flour provide essential nutrients like iron and folic acid, you don't get those in many gluten-free foods.

Another important worry: Many gluten-free products contain rice flour or other rice-based ingredients. In tests of rice and rice products in 2012, researchers found that most contain arsenic, often at worrisome levels.

One more disadvantage to going gluten free: Nearly all the gluten-free foods *Consumer Reports* purchased were more expensive than a regular counterpart.

If you are truly gluten sensitive, then I recommend you explore MayoClinic.org and WebMD.com. Both have useful pages related to gluten-free dieting, which can help you adapt my Tighten Your Tummy eating plan to eliminate gluten. Basically, both Web sites advise the following:

1. These foods are allowed: beans, seeds, nuts, eggs, meat, poultry, fish, vegetables, fruits, and most dairy products.
2. These foods should be avoided: wheat, rye, and barley, as well as drinks containing malt flavoring or malt vinegar. Most beer is out.
3. Be careful with these foods (unless they are labeled "gluten free"): breads, cakes, pies, candies, cereals (except those made of corn), french fries, processed meats, and salad dressings.
4. Watch for cross-contamination: This usually happens during the manufacturing process, if the equipment is used to mix and make a variety of products. In other words, cross-contamination occurs when gluten-free foods come in contact with foods that contain gluten, even the remains that are left in various mixing machines. Check carefully the actual ingredient list on the product. Be aware that the same cross-contamination also can occur in restaurants or in your own home. Ask questions and be prepared to walk away and not buy.
5. Going gluten free is not easy: It means giving up many staples, such as breads, cereals, and pasta. And generally, people who

benefit from eating gluten free need to stick with the eating style for life. But it is getting easier to find 100 percent gluten-free alternatives.

Your goal with gluten-free dieting is to still keep the same daily calorie levels, size, and frequency of meals.

Lower Abs

Q: I think my lower abs are weakest and need the most work. Does your program target them?

A: All the recommended floor exercises involve your lower abdominal muscles. But you won't feel the kind of burn from an abdominal exercise in the lower area the way you will in the upper area. Here are the reasons why.

- The largest section of your abdominal muscles is high on your waist, under your rib cage, not beneath your navel. You almost always feel abdominal strain most in the mass of the muscle toward the origin.

- The long, paired rectus abdominis muscles originate under your rib cage and insert into your pelvis. But when these muscles get near the region of your navel, they actually plunge through an opening in the horizontally crossing transverse abdominis muscles. The transverse abdominis, which lies on top of the insertion point of the rectus abdominis, tends to reduce the sensitivity of the deeper rectus abdominis.

- Muscles begin their contractile process at the ends, where the tendons attach to the bones, and move gradually toward the center. Thus, to work the portion of the rectus that inserts on your pelvis, you have to move slowly at the extended position of each exercise. Work diligently at mastering the 15-15-15 protocol and you should be able to generate additional feeling into the lower-abdominal area—especially as the involved muscles get stronger.

Muscle Turning to Fat

Q: If I build several pounds of muscle on your program and then stop exercising, will the muscle turn to fat?

A: Absolutely not. Muscles are muscles, and fat is fat. There is no way one can turn into the other.

Muscle is composed of 70 percent water, 22 percent proteins, and 7 percent lipids or fat. Fat is 15 percent water, 6 percent proteins, and 79 percent lipids. So, like an apple and an orange, muscle and fat, though related in composition, are chemically and genetically different. If you stop strength training, you will gradually lose muscle mass. With less calorie-burning muscle on your body, you can add fat stores. But the muscle itself will never turn into fat.

The Truth about Cellulite

Q: I'm plagued by cellulite around my lower belly, hips, and upper thighs. You haven't mentioned anything about how to combat it. How can I smooth out my cellulite?

A: The reason I have not specifically mentioned cellulite is because the word itself is not scientific. The word was created over 50 years ago and popularized by Nicole Ronsard in her 1973 book, *Cellulite: Those Lumps, Bumps, and Bulges You Couldn't Lose Before.* (The paperback version of this book is still available.)

Although there is no such scientific term as *cellulite*, the condition to which the word refers does exist. Most middle-aged women have thick layers of fat on their buttocks and upper thighs. What's referred to as cellulite is subcutaneous (below the skin) adipose tissue just like any common body fat. It is nothing more than stored fat. The dimpled effect is caused by the fibers of connective tissue in the area, which lose their elasticity with age. The overlying skin attached to these fibers then contracts. If the size of the encased fat cells does not shrink proportionately, a kind of overall dimpling occurs on the surface of the skin.

In her book, Ronsard discusses a six-part plan to combat cellulite. Briefly the components are (1) diet, (2) proper elimination, (3) breathing and oxygenation, (4) exercise, (5) massage, and (6) relaxation. While each of the components plays some role in removing fat, none of her specific details are close to the most efficient way to get rid of a woman's fatty lumps and bulges.

Here's the truth about cellulite:

- The dimpling effect of the fat on the overlying skin is caused by the combination of overfatness, loss of muscular size and strength, and the natural aging of the connective tissue.

- Women store several times more fat on their hips and thighs than do men. Much of this is related to hormones and the ability to conceive children.

- Fat cannot be massaged, perspired, relaxed, soaked, flushed, compressed, or dissolved out of the human body.

- The treatment for dimpled fatty deposits is a twofold approach:

  - *You must reduce the size of the fat cells by dieting.*
  - *You must increase the size and strength of the large muscle groups that compose the hips and thighs.*

While the Tighten Your Tummy program will certainly help the condition, a broader program that involves more negative-accentuated exercise for the lower body is found in my book *The Body Fat Breakthrough*.

Where Does Lost Fat Go?

Q: **I've been through your program. I lost 20 pounds of fat, and I keep wondering, where does all that fat go when it leaves my body?**

A: That's a great question. The answer involves a little chemistry, but I'll try to keep it simple. You should understand by now that fat translates to calories, and calories are units of heat energy.

Heat emerges from your body in three ways—through your lungs, skin, and urine. Years ago, Albert Einstein and other scientists proved that you can't create or destroy energy. You can only transfer it. Thus, when you lose fat, you transfer the energy stored in fat cells out of your body and into the environment. Once in the environment, it is available for use by other living organisms and by the environment. With each use, heat energy is once again transferred, and the cycle continues endlessly. That's the simple answer.

A slightly different response can be found in the *British Medical Journal* (December 16, 2014). In a study of how energy is metabolized, researchers Ruben Meerman and Andrew Brown traced the pathways of atoms of energy exiting the body. The complete oxidation of a single triglyceride molecule involves many enzymes and biochemical steps, but after lengthy calculations, Meerman and Brown concluded that triglycerides stored in fat cells are primarily excreted by the lungs through respiration. Stored fat is unlocked through chemical reactions to power your body, including during exercise, and it exits the body as your exhaled breath.

According to Meerman and Brown, when a person loses 20 pounds of fat (triglyceride), 16.8 pounds are exhaled as warm carbon dioxide (CO_2), and the remaining 3.2 pounds are excreted as warm water (H_2O), primarily in the urine and sweat.

But, the researchers caution, body fat does not shrink quickly. Applying the standard reduced-calorie eating/increased-calorie exercising formula, they recommend 1 pound of fat loss per week. Thus, it would take 20 weeks for the average person to lose 20 pounds of fat.

On the other hand, my Tighten Your Tummy formula speeds up the fat-loss process to the degree that each of my 41 women lost an average of 2.5 pounds of fat each week, which equates to 20 pounds of fat loss in 8 weeks. That's 2.5 times the fat loss in 40 percent of the time suggested by Meerman and Brown.

Why are my fat-loss results so much better and more efficient than those recommended by Meerman and Brown? Because besides having a reduced-calorie diet, my plan involves at least four other fat-loss factors:

- Negative-accentuated exercise to trigger muscle growth and raise metabolism

- Skin emphasis (radiation, conduction, convection, evaporation) to maximize heat release

- Extra sleep in a cool environment to assist recovery and expand fat burning

- Superhydration to increase urine production and synergize the fat-loss process

Sickness and Training

Q: **If I'm feeling sick, should I still try to squeeze in a negative-accentuated workout?**

A: No. Both illness and negative-accentuated training make heavy demands on your recovery ability. Continuing to exercise during periods of illness retards your recovery. It can actually aggravate the illness. So use your illness as extra incentive to rest, rest, rest. As a rule, you should rest one day for every day you were sick before returning to your negative-accentuated routine. And when you start up again, you should exercise at a lower level of intensity.

Holiday Guidelines

Q: **I always have trouble staying on a diet during the holidays, and I fear I'll regain some of my lost fat. Do you have any advice for ways to avoid all these festive calories?**

A: You are wise to want to be prepared. The average woman in the United States gains approximately 5 pounds between Thanksgiving and January 2. It comes down to being disciplined, but here are some actions that should help you:

- Be conscious more than ever of the value of drinking ice water. One gallon each day will work wonders to keep you full and stall cravings for high-calorie snacks.

- Take 30-minute after-dinner walks regularly (get up and get out quickly—you'll eat less).

- Cut up a lot of vegetables and have them handy for snacks. For parties, fill a relish tray with cut vegetables and fruits and use fat-free yogurt for dip.

- Perfect a couple of low-calorie delicacies to take to parties. One woman in my Tighten Your Tummy test panel even took one of her favorite Lean Cuisine dinners to a Christmas party, cooked, and ate it—instead of consuming a higher-calorie meal.

- Eliminate alcohol altogether. Besides the waistline savings, you'll drive home safer.

- Say no to others urging you to eat against your will.

- Practice staying cool. Dress lighter than normal. Avoid wearing a hat.

- Buy a tight-fitting New Year's Eve outfit and try it on twice a week.

- Give your low-calorie dinners the trappings of elegance—good china, candlelight, and soft music.

- Plan special events that do not revolve around food.

- Sleep more.

- Follow up by keeping a daily journal of your eating, water drinking, and exercising.

A Tall Woman, a Short Woman

Q: On your Tighten Your Tummy program, does a really tall woman or a really short woman have to do anything differently?

A: Probably not, unless you are taller than 6 feet or shorter than 5 feet. My tallest test panelist was Barbara Trombetta at 6 feet, and the shortest was Pam Waters at 5 feet. They both followed the same eating plan, and each lost pounds and inches within the range of average.

If you are over 6 feet tall, then you have more surface area (skin) available to the environment—as a result, you'll have a higher metabolism. You'll probably need an extra 100 calories added to your daily requirements. Over 6 weeks, instead of applying 1,000, 1,200, and 1,100 calories at 2-week transitions, increase the calories by 100 to 1,100, 1,300, and 1,200.

On the other hand, if you are under 5 feet, the opposite is true: You have less surface area (skin) available to the environment, and your metabolism is lower than average. Perhaps 50 fewer calories per day would work better for you. Try the following levels: 950, 1,150, and 1,050 calories per day. (Note: As I state in Chapter 6, I don't recommend going below 1,000 calories a day. But with certain women who are under 5 feet tall, I make exceptions.)

Homemade Breakfast Shake

Q: **I like an occasional meal-replacement shake for breakfast, but I can't find the two brands you recommend [in Chapter 15]. Any suggestions on how I can make my own at home?**

A: Here's a recipe for one of my favorite breakfast shakes. Weighing in at approximately 300 calories, it's a good source of quality carbohydrates and protein, and is delicious and satisfying.

Banana Malt Shake

8 ounces 2% milk

1 medium banana

1 egg white, cooked

1 tablespoon malted milk powder

1 tablespoon honey or brown sugar

¼ teaspoon vanilla extract

Dash of ground cinnamon or nutmeg

Combine all the ingredients in a blender. Cover and blend on medium speed until smooth. Instead of the banana, you may substitute 100 calories of various fruits, such as strawberries, blueberries, or peaches.

Keep Cool

Q: **You mentioned in Chapter 7 that keeping your body cool will help you burn more calories. Do you have any additional tips for doing that?**

A: Here are some practices that will assist you in losing more calories by staying cool.

- Dress cooler and lighter at work.

- Take off your coat sooner and keep it off longer.

- Select short sleeves more often.

- Don't wear a hat.

- Turn down the thermostat.

- Leave off your socks at home, or go barefoot more often.

- Try to remain uncomfortably cool throughout the day and allow your skin's heating mechanism time to adjust.

- Negative-train in a cooler environment, if possible.

- Wear light, well-ventilated clothing when you exercise.

- Avoid sauna, steam, and whirlpool baths, as they cause excessive heat accumulation.

- Take cold showers after exercise.

- Place cold compresses on the back of your neck.

- Sleep cooler.

- Wean yourself from electric blankets and flannel sheets in the winter.

Ideal Percent Body Fat

Q: What do you consider the ideal body fat percentage for a woman?

A: The ideal percent body fat changes slightly as a woman gets older. At age 20, I like to see most women at 18 percent or below. At 25, 19 percent is the number, and at 30, it goes up to 20 percent. There's a slight increase with each 5-year period. So at age 35, it's 20.5 percent, then 21 percent at age 40, 21.5 percent at age 45, and 22 percent at age 50. At 55 years of age, it's 22.5 percent, and it goes up to 23 percent at age 60. After age 60, the percent remains at 23.

These recommendations are based on thousands of body fat measurements I've taken using the Lange Skinfold Caliper over the past 40 years. There are many different ways to measure body fat. The most accurate and expensive is DEXA scan, which involves taking a full dual x-ray of your body. Water displacement, which requires submersion in water, is expensive, too. A device called the Bod Pod calculates body fat percentage by using air displacement to measure your body mass, volume, and density. Body fat scales send an electrical current through your body, but they are highly inaccurate. I still believe the proper use of the Lange caliper is the simplest and more effective way to determine percent body fat—and also the best way to estimate muscle gain by subtracting a woman's weight loss from her fat loss.

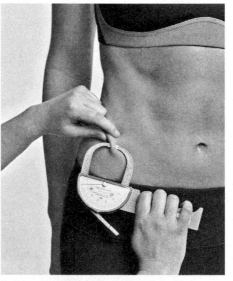

To determine body fat percentage, I use a Lange Skinfold Caliper to measure thickness of a pinch of skin and fat at three spots on the body—the triceps, hip (shown), and thigh. The numbers are added and compared to a scientific table, which produces a percent body fat reading.

Of the 41 women in the Tighten Your Tummy test panel, the ones pictured in this book who achieved the lowest percent body fat were:

1. Marlene Hill: 15.4 percent
2. Sarah Darden: 16.7 percent
3. Brianna Kramer: 17 percent
4. Sara Smith: 17.1 percent
5. Denise Rodriguez: 17.3 percent
6. Vera Sodek: 19.6 percent
7. Elena Mavrodieva: 19.8 percent

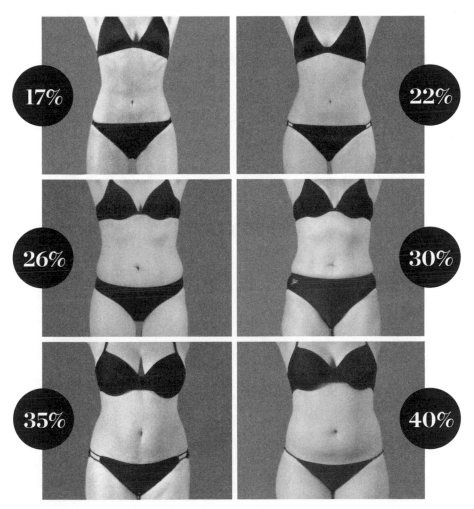

This grid provides a closeup comparison of six women's midsections at various amounts of body fat, from a low of 17 percent body fat to high of 40 percent.

chapter

20

Best Tips for Success!

Failproof Your Weight Loss with Secrets from the Tighten Your Tummy Test Panelists

You now have the blueprint to tighten your tummy, get into great shape, and improve your health. As you've learned, losing weight and building muscle/fitness/good health is a process. It takes effort. It's not always easy to stick to a healthy meal plan when you are busy and the drive-thru seems like the most convenient solution. A bad day at home or work might make a glass of Chardonnay or a pint of rocky road ice cream look very comforting.

The Tighten Your Tummy test panelists at Gainesville Health & Fitness have been there. They've experienced the program and its challenges—some of them twice! They know the pitfalls and tough spots, and they've learned how to overcome them. They have, through trial and error and sheer determination, found ways to hurdle the daunting obstacles that stand in their way. And they have been rewarded for their dedication and ingenuity with leaner, fitter bodies.

One example is Katie Smith, an amazing woman. In 40 years of working with clients trying to lose weight, I've never had a woman lose as much as Katie. In 18 weeks, she lost more than 60 pounds of fat and 25 inches off her waist! Katie and her friend, Joan Cortez, were an inspiration throughout the program. Both retired schoolteachers, Katie and Joan set an example for fellow dieters and, through the kindness and firm discipline that marked their careers as educators, motivated and mentored their friends throughout the program.

Seeing how effective their examples were, I asked all the test panelists to share their best tips, hints, secrets, and strategies for success with you. When the going gets tough, just flip through this chapter. There's a tip to stay on track in any—and every—situation. It's like having a team of experienced mentors with you every step of the way!

Sticking to the Program

Always have a plan. A road map or GPS is helpful when driving to a place you haven't been before. The same is true when your destination is a new body. Each morning when Katie got out of bed, she had a schedule to go by. She knew what she was going to do and when to do it. Each night, she aimed to head to bed with a fully checked to-do list and would use it to outline the following day's tasks.

Expect imperfection. Katie kept her journal for 126 consecutive days! It wasn't flawless—some days a task would be left unchecked—but perfection isn't the point; it's just a goal. "Don't be discouraged when something pops up," says Katie. "Just adjust and keep moving through the day." Need inspiration for your first day? Check out my wife Jeanenne's journal entry on page xiv.

Bring backup. Eating away from home can make sticking to a meal plan challenging. "If I knew I wasn't going to make it home during the day, I made sandwiches and packed them in a small ice chest along with snacks like yogurt, apples, or almonds and a jug of ice water," says Vera Sodek. "This made it easy to stick to the diet and not worry about returning home at a certain time for a meal or snack."

Adjusting to Smaller Portions

Recognize real meal sizes. "In the beginning, I would look at my meal and say 'Is this it?'" says Denise Rodriguez. But she and many of the test panelists found there is something to be learned from the puzzle-like packing of frozen entrées: A 300-calorie meal can be filling, delicious, and include all the nutrients you need for a balanced meal. "Eating the frozen meals really helps you 'eyeball' what an acceptable portion looks like later," says Pam Waters, who lost 18 pounds on the program.

And although some packaged food gets a bad rap for poor taste or quality, you can trust in these carefully vetted suggestions from the Tighten Your Tummy team. "They taste good, and the calories are the same as the program's guidelines," notes Joan Cortez. Plus, she adds, several brands use whole grains and freeze-fresh ingredients.

Here are some of the test panelists' favorites.

Amy's Light & Lean Italian Vegetable Pizza

Applegate Naturals Chicken & Apple Breakfast Sausage Patties

Barilla Italian Entrees Tomato & Basil Whole Grain Penne

Earthbound Farm Organic PowerMeal Bowl Blueberry & Quinoa & Baby Spinach

Healthy Choice Café Steamers Tortellini Primavera Parmesan

Lean Cuisine Culinary Collection Lemon Pepper Fish

Lean Cuisine Culinary Collection Orange Chicken

Lean Cuisine Alfredo Pasta with Chicken and Broccoli

Lundberg Family Farms Organic Wild Porcini Mushroom Whole Grain Rice & Wild Rice

Saffron Road Bibimbop with Tofu & Brown Rice

Dealing with Cravings

Find smart swaps. If you're craving something crunchy, try baby carrots and hummus. Must have potato chips? Cut whole grain pitas into triangles and bake them. If it's cheese and crackers you want, swap out the cheese for wasabi spread. "The robust, hot flavor really gets your attention," says Sarah Darden. Don't have wasabi handy? Try horseradish or hot sauce. Capsaicin, the chemical in peppers that gives them their bite, can actually help you lose weight by speeding up your heart rate. Studies have shown that eating a single spicy meal can boost your metabolism by up to 25 percent, with the spike in calorie burning lasting for up to 3 hours after you finish eating.

Keep busy. Occupying your hands and your brain can keep both out of the cookie jar. "Take up some of the Pinterest projects you have been pinning," advises Jennifer MacCallum, 34, a mother of four children who lost 34 pounds of fat in 12 weeks. Work in the yard. Start a scrapbook. Knit. Anything that takes your mind off hunger can help.

Skipping Dessert

Fill up first. If you always end a meal with dessert, break the habit by eating to satisfaction. Amping up your entrée can help. Katie recommends sautéing 1 cup of cabbage (slaw type) and an onion in 1 tablespoon of coconut oil. Add the mix to your frozen entrée for a heartier meal. "It was just enough that I felt more full after eating it slowly," says Katie. Another way to feel fuller: Change your perspective by eating on smaller plates, says Laura Morrow, who lost 21 pounds in 6 weeks on the Tighten Your Tummy program. "It makes your plate look full!"

Pack your plate. Load up on fresh fruits, says Marlene Hill. "I like to add a lot of different fruits, vegetables, and seeds to my salads to make them more filling," she says. And if sweet temptation still strikes after a meal, she keeps her healthiest options within arm's reach. "I always keep a fruit bowl packed with seasonal fruit on my dining table," says Marlene.

Have a low-cal sweet. Test panelists have used all sorts of substitutes for after-dinner sweet treats. Give these a try:

- Suck on a sugar-free hard candy.

- Chew a chewable vitamin C supplement tablet.

- Have a small piece of whole fruit.

- Savor one spoonful of chocolate ice cream. Just one.

- Blend fresh fruit with $\frac{1}{2}$ cup of low-fat yogurt or kefir.

- Eat a small square of bitter dark chocolate.

- Swipe on a mint-scented lip balm.

- Suck on an ice cube made from sugar-free limeade.

- Take a dip in a scented bubble bath, or fill your home with candles that are cinnamon bun- or strawberry smoothie-scented. You'll get a waft of something heavenly sweet without having to indulge the extra calories.

Drinking All That Water!

I really like Jeanenne's tip for keeping track of her water consumption (detailed in Chapter 8): She moved rubber bands up and down her tumbler every time she refilled her water bottle. Test panelists found other ways to make drinking a gallon of ice water a day easier.

Keep it handy. If your water bottle is always within reach, you'll be more likely to sip all day long, say test panelists. Fill up a large tumbler with ice water and keep it on your desk at work. Take one to the gym. Leave one in your car. Make it a habit to drink a tumbler of ice water before every meal and snack.

Add flavorings. "Add slices of lemons or limes to your ice water for taste variety," Joan suggests. Or try calorie-free or low-calorie flavor packets. "Slender Sticks by NOW are awesome," she says. "They're sweetened with stevia, and one packet contains only 15 calories!" Try crystallized lime packets, like True Lime (truecitrus.com, $4.99).

Practice feeling full. As you've learned, water helps you feel fuller. Reminding yourself that water is your secret weight-loss weapon may make it easier to meet your daily quota. "Whenever I felt hungry, I reached for my water bottle and sipped a lot of water at once to feel full," says Barbara Trombetta. "Doing so got me to the next snack or meal." Nannette Carnes says, "I knew that the more water I drank, the less hungry I would feel. I also knew that drinking ice-cold water would burn more fat."

Eating Out and Eating with Others

BYO! What do you do when dining with friends at restaurants or at parties? The temptation to join the party can be tremendous unless you prepare ahead of time. Barbara owes her 15-pound fat loss to her new beverage of choice: LaCroix sparkling flavored water. "At happy hour, I just poured a glass or two of it in a wine or champagne glass," says Barbara. "The seltzer bubbles made me feel like I was drinking something special." At dinner parties, ask your host if you can bring a dish you can share and savor with friends. "I always took my own food to parties or dinners," says Joan. "Travel with your own party in a bag and remember: The veggie tray is great, but not with dips!"

    Research the menu. "The most important thing to do before eating at a restaurant is to get on the Internet and look up the menu and nutritional value of each meal," says Joan. Plan your order before arriving and ask the waiter to hold off on bread or chips for the table.

    Cut it in half. Restaurants are notorious for big plates and big portions. "As soon as my order comes out, I divide it in half down the plate with a fork," says Angela Choate. "Halving your order once it's out keeps the idea of portion control fresh on your mind before you dig in."

    Play it safe. Can't find the menu online? Stick with salad, says Pam: "I order mine with oil, vinegar, lemon on the side, and request broiled fish or chicken." Most places will accommodate what you want. Just be sure to ask for your protein sauce-free and think of the plate as a pie chart—50 percent carbohydrates, 25 percent protein, and 25 percent fat. When you're unsure if a half-size is small enough, keep your order simple, says Angela: "I order a cup of soup and side salad with dressing on the side."

    Dodge the dessert tray. When everyone around you seems to want something sweet, pop a mint in your mouth, says Denise. "It keeps your mouth busy and your mind preoccupied while everyone's eating." If the craving persists, indulge your sweet tooth by savoring a slice of fresh fruit or small square of dark chocolate instead.

(continued on page 218)

TRAIN YOUR TASTE BUDS TO HELP YOU LOSE WEIGHT

Craving-beating tips from a Tighten Your Tummy coach and dental hygienist

Lydia Maree is the best dental hygienist *and* assistant fitness coach I've had the opportunity to work with. Over the past 20+ years, she's kept my smile shining, and more recently, she's helped me plan, organize, train, and assess the success of all my weight-loss project test panelists over the past four years.

So I asked Lydia to share some tips regarding an often-neglected, but all-too-important body part to think about when you're dieting—your mouth! Training your taste buds will help support your weight loss and give those pearly whites a glossy finish.

"Having a clean mouth reduces the desire to eat because most people don't want to mask that just-brushed freshness feeling," says Lydia.

Next time you feel a craving or feel that you are still hungry and may overeat, try one or two of these proven strategies to dull the urge to eat:

- Floss your teeth with different-flavored flosses (mint, bubble gum, cinnamon, cherry, or grape).
- Brush your teeth with different-flavored toothpastes (bubble gum, spearmint, wintergreen, or cherry).
- Scrape or brush your tongue with a toothbrush.
- Have a stick of low-calorie or sugar-free gum when you feel the onset of hunger.
- Sprinkle cinnamon instead of sugar or sugar replacements. The antioxidants in the spice stabilize blood sugar and slow digestion.

- Suck on a sugar-free peppermint. Several studies attribute physical and psychological benefits to peppermint, and some dieters swear that the minty taste helps them ward off hunger pains. For a similar effect, try dabbing a few drops of essential peppermint oil on your tongue.

- Close your eyes and *imagine* yourself eating the food that you are craving . . . very slowly. Think about the texture of the food and how it makes you feel afterward. Practice this visualization exercise repeatedly to reduce your cravings.

- Change up your food choices to alter the textures of foods that you eat to reduce hunger pains. Go from crunchy to smooth to sticky to tacky and alternate the patterns frequently. Textures of food become very important to dieters, so vary your choices to improve your chances of success.

- Use flavored lip balm like grape or cherry that you can taste when you lick your lips to reduce cravings.

- Chew your food well to benefit your mouth beyond the tasty-on-the-tongue factor. Not only does food taste better the more you chew, chewing also increases saliva production, helping to digest bacteria that can lead to plaque buildup. The more you break your food down in your mouth, the less work there is for your stomach and intestines. This can mean less gas and bloating and better elimination. Your intestines also have an easier time pulling micronutrients out of well-chewed food than big chunks, which provides your body with more vitamins, minerals, antioxidants, and amino acids.

Making Time to Walk a Mile

Invite others. "Walking after dinner became family time," says Denise. Every evening after dinner, Denise, her husband, and their 2-year-old daughter would take a stroll around their neighborhood and pass the time by talking about their day. "It actually really brought us together," says Denise. Reserving her walks as family time helped Denise unwind from busy days with two of her biggest supporters. "We still make time for walks today," she says.

Unwind. "I made my walks part of my day to meditate," says Angela. "I left the dogs at home and made time for myself instead." So take a break to walk a mile in your own shoes. "It was personal time that I could use to reflect." As Angela looped the cul-de-sac in her neighborhood, she says she focused on how good it felt to be outside, on sipping her water, and on what she'd accomplished that day.

Walking in Bad Weather

Go window-shopping. Many of the Tighten Your Tummy test panelists had the pleasure of living in sunny Florida. But when the skies were cloudy or temperatures dipped, they still made time for walks. "Walk the mall!" says Angela. If you don't have a gym membership, a big mall easily serves as a stand-in for treadmills on a rainy day.

March in place. "If the weather is bad, I will walk in place at home," says Nellie Otero. "And if I happen to miss a day, I drop the guilt and pick it up the next day."

Switch it up! When you're bored with the same routine, add more variety by biking your usual walking route, says Joan. Another alternative if you have joint pain: Try swimming instead of walking. "I swam for 30 minutes at the gym by doing laps or treading water," she says.

Catching More Z's

Set your bedtime. Denise took a cue from her 2-year-old on how to sleep more soundly: Stick to your bedtime. "I make sure that everything is accomplished before dinnertime," says Denise. "Every night, I know it's dinner, walking, get ready for bed. Anything I can't accomplish before dinner can wait till tomorrow morning."

Turn off the TV. Open a book or a journal instead. "Journaling before bed helps get rid of restless thoughts," says Nellie. What's more, that blue hue can mess with your melatonin levels, causing you to have trouble nodding off and even more trouble sleeping soundly. If silence doesn't suit you, try meditating to music. "I like Virtual Gastric Band Hypnosis (iTunes, $6.99)," says Joan. "Each night you listen to lectures with a soothing voice about making better choices for eating. It sinks in because it is repeated over and over. It is so soothing you drift off to sleep."

Backsliding

Beat diet boredom! By the end of the program, Melissa Jones expressed that eating the same foods day in and day out was making her less interested in sticking with the diet. She made a few small tweaks before it was too late. When a bagel and cream cheese starts to feel stale, try a muffin with the same number of calories. The day your baby carrots and hummus don't cut it, try ants on a log instead. The subtle changes will be just enough to revive your taste buds without stifling your progress.

Set a short-term goal. While you're working toward a long-term weight-loss goal, it's important to set smaller, achievable benchmarks to keep you motivated and boost your confidence along the way, says Lynn James. Weekly weigh-ins will keep you on track to see how your weight progress is going, but snapping pictures will help you see how the program tones your physique. "Before-and-after pictures will definitely keep you on your toes," says Lynn. When you set a short-term goal, make it realistic but tough enough that you have to fully focus on the program to achieve it. "If you look at the program as 'Oh, it's only 2 weeks,' it really puts things in perspective," says Lynn. "It's such a short time, it really pushes you to say 'I can do it!' and actually do it."

Look ahead. Don't dwell on an error; just start back the next day, says Nellie. "It does not have to be all or nothing." Learn from the misstep and move on. The less time you spend worrying about a bump in the road, the more time you have to pave over mistakes and move forward even faster than before.

Raid your closet. Ready to keep weight off for good? Clean out your pantry—and your closets, say the panelists. Laura lost her weight by clearing tempting foods from her fridge and kitchen cabinets. "Get rid of them, or at least keep them out of your sight and reach," says Laura. Katie gave away her old clothes and revamped her wardrobe with slimmer-fitting clothing as incentive to maintain her weight loss.

Phone a friend. Recruit a partner to take on the program with you, or use this diet as an incentive to make new friends walking or at the gym.

A MAGIC BULLET THAT CAN HELP YOU SUCCEED

IT IS SO STRAIGHTFORWARD THAT IT'S easy to take for granted. Among the women who saw the greatest results in the Tighten Your Tummy test panels, a critical concept emerged. Each of these women, the best of my test panelists, Roxanne Dybevick, Katie Smith, Joan Cortez, Jennifer MacCallum, and Marlene Hill displayed it.

What was that one thing?

CONSISTENCY. Day after day, each of these women followed the program (and each new set of instructions) with rock-solid consistency.

There was no need to mope around directionless for days or weeks—waiting for enthusiasm to appear. These women used the simplicity of the program to stay on course and produce amazing results.

Katie Smith, who lost 62.73 pounds of fat and 25.6 inches off her waist, said it better than anyone: "I was adrift in the ocean in a boat that could not navigate itself . . . hoping to have someone help. The Tighten Your Tummy program rescued me. I was given the tools to repair my vessel. But consistent effort every day made all the difference."

Developing relationships with fellow dieters will keep you en route to success and help you maintain your weight after you've met your goal. "Share phone numbers and e-mails with them so that if you are struggling, they can help you get through your problems," says Brianna Kramer. "Chances are, they are probably going through the same issues, and it's a lot easier to keep going when you know you're not alone."

I want to thank all the Tighten Your Tummy test panelists who shared their hints, tips, and advice. Follow their lead and you'll reach your goal.

Some women like Nellie Otero, Laura Morrow, and Pam Waters followed the Tighten Your Tummy diet exactly as it is presented in this book. Other women like Katie Smith, Lynn James, and Angela Choate made adaptations to fit it into their lifestyles. But the common theme among these women was consistency.

Whatever category you're in, the correct diet is a valuable start. Combined with the other proven practices— superhydration, negative-accentuated strength training, the inner-ab vacuum, and 8½ hours of sleep each night—it's a challenging but doable program that can transform your body and your life.

APPLY, ADAPT, BELIEVE, and most of all, be CONSISTENT and you'll achieve a tighter tummy, too.

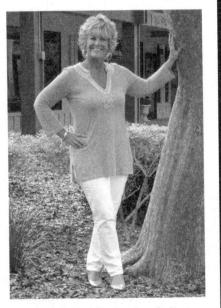

Katie Smith and her brand-new body

bibliography

Bercsheid, Ellen, and Pamela C. Regan. *The Psychology of Interpersonal Relationships*. New York: Person Prentice Hall, 2005.

Boschmann, Michael, and others. "Water-Induced Thermogenesis," *Journal of Clinical Endocrinology & Metabolism* 88: 6015–6019, 2003.

Darden, Ellington. *The Body Fat Breakthrough*. New York: Rodale, 2014.

————. *Two Weeks to a Tighter Tummy*. Dallas: Taylor, 1992.

————. *The Nautilus Diet*. Boston: Little, Brown, 1987.

Davis, J. Mark, and others. "Weight Control and Calorie Expenditure: Thermogenesis Effects of Pre-Prandial Exercise," *Addictive Behaviors* 14: 347–351, 1989.

Dreisbach, Shaun. "How Do You Feel About Your Body," *Glamour*, November 2014: 137–143.

Elliot, Danielle. "The Doctor Who Coaches Athletes on Sleep," *The Atlantic*, April 23, 2014.

Ford, Earl S., and others. "Trends in Mean Waist Circumference and Abdominal Obesity Among US Adults, 1999–2012," *Journal of the American Medical Association* 312:1151–1153, 2014.

Gibbons, Ann. "The Evolution of Diet," *National Geographic* 226: 34–65, September 2014.

Heymsfield, Steven B., and others. "Evolving Concepts on Adjusting Human Resting Energy Expenditure Measurements for Body Size," *Obesity Reviews* 13:1001–1014, 2012.

Johns Hopkins University. *The Johns Hopkins Family Health Book*. New York: HarperCollins, 1998.

Lassek, Will, and others. "Eternal Curves," *Psychology Today*, July 3, 2012.

Levinovitz, Alan. *The Gluten Lie and Other Myths About What You Eat*. New York: Regan Arts, 2015.

Mah, Cheri D., and others. "The Effects of Sleep Extension on Athletic Performance of College Basketball Players," *Sleep* 34: 943–950, 2011.

Meerman, Ruben, and Andrew Brown. "When Somebody Loses Weight, Where Does the Fat Go?" *British Medical Journal*, December 16, 2014.

Nedeitcheva, Arlet V., and others. "Insufficient Sleep Undermines Dietary Efforts to Reduce Adiposity," *Annals of Internal Medicine* 153: 435–441, 2010.

Pollock, M. L., and others. "Measurement of Cardiorespiratory and Body Composition in the Clinical Setting," *Comprehensive Therapy* 6:12–27, 1980.

Roig, M., and others. "The Effects of Eccentric Versus Concentric Resistance Training on Muscle Strength and Mass in Healthy Adults: A Systematic Review with Meta-Analyses," *British Journal of Sports Medicine* 43:556–568, 2009.

Sartori, Robert, and others. "BMP Signaling Controls Muscle Mass," *Nature Genetics* 45:1309–1318, 2013.

Schuler, Lou. "The Truth about Raspberry Ketones, Green Coffee Bean Extract, and Garcinia Cambogia," *Menshealth.com*, June 24, 2014.

Singh, Devendra. "Adaptive Significance of Female Physical Attractiveness: Role of Waist-to-Hip Ratio," *Journal of Personality and Social Psychology* 65: 293–307, 1993.

Sizer, Francis, and Ellie Whitney. *Nutrition Concepts & Controversies* (paperback 12th edition). Belmont, CA: Wadsworth, Cengage Learning, 2012.

Spalding, Kirsty L., and others. "Dynamics of Fat Cell Turnover," *Nature* 453: 783–787, 2008.

"The Truth about Gluten," *Consumer Reports* 80: 36–40, January 2015.

Whitten, Ari, and Wade Smith. *The Low Carb Myth*. Lexington, KY: Archangel Ink, 2015.

Winett, Richard A., and Ralph N. Carpinelli. "Potential Health-Related Benefits of Resistance Training," *Preventive Medicine* 33: 503–513, 2001.

acknowledgments

I want to thank some important people, who had a positive influence on the writing of this book.

The 41 women from **Gainesville Health & Fitness**, which made up my Tighten Your Tummy test panel, were a superb group of trainees. They absorbed the program for 42 consecutive days, and the average results were the most outstanding I've ever been associated with.

Roxanne Dybevick, Katie Smith, Jennifer MacCallum, Nellie Otero, Mary Dees, and **Joan Cortez,** as members of the test panel, showed great leadership skills. Their actions encouraged me to challenge and direct the group *intensely* to reach their goals. The Latin phrase *E pluribus unum,* or "Out of many, one," succinctly captures the determination of this diverse group of 41 women. This motto soon became a motivating force throughout all of our lives.

My daughter, **Sarah**, who exceeded my expectations for getting her body in top shape. I am so pleased that you responded to my training. Yes, Sarah, we did it!

My wife, **Jeanenne**, who kicked a protruding belly in the mouth—and inspired me to plan and follow through with the Tighten Your Tummy course.

Joe Cirulli, owner of Gainesville Health & Fitness, and his experienced staff and colleagues, namely: **Lydia Maree, Jim Lennon, Ann Raulerson, Pam Harrison,** and **Mike Spillane.** You smoothed out numerous rough edges for me and I appreciate your consistent work ethic.

Don Brown, who invented the Ab-Roller Evolution, for his support and marketing intelligence and savvy.

Jeff Csatari, executive editor of Men's Health and Women's Health books at Rodale, who is the best editor I've ever worked with. Thank you, Jeff, for sharing your talents.

Also, thanks to **Nancy N. Bailey** and **Gillian Francella** for their attention to detail during the production process.

Mitch Mandel of Rodale for taking the great photos of Sarah, and **Carol Angstadt** for her impressive art direction and book design.

Amy C. King of Rodale for the most attention-getting book cover I've ever seen. Your bright pink concept was unexpected and similar to fireworks at midnight. Thank you, Amy, for working so smoothly outside and inside the box.

The "After Photos" Show

The Tighten Your Tummy program transformed their bodies and improved their lives.

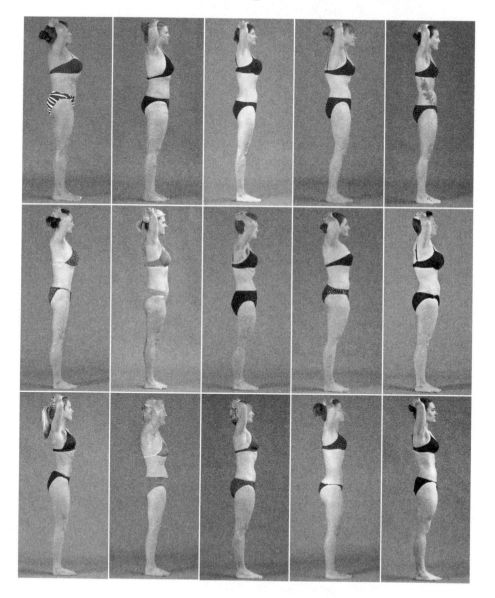

Now it's your turn to join them.

index

Bold page references indicate pictures.
Underscored page references indicate boxed text and tables.

A

Abdominal muscles
  Ab Roller exercises for
    forward crunch, 102–3, **103**
    obliques crunch, 104–5, **105**
    V-crunch, 106–7, **107**
  defined, 10, 35–36
  exercises for
    forward crunch, 84–87, **85–87**
    obliques crunch, 88–89, **89**
    V-crunch, 90–91, **91**
  lower, toning, 200
Abdominal obesity zone, 17
Ab Roller Evolution, 100
Ab Roller exercises, 100–115
  dumbbell curl, 112–13, **113**
  dumbbell overhead press, 114–15,
    115
  forward crunch, 102–3, **103**
  obliques crunch, 104–5, **105**
  pushups, 108–9, **109**
  squats, 110–11, **111**
  V-crunch, 106–7, **107**
Actresses and models, 3, 5–6
Adiponectin, 34
Adrenaline, 33, 38, 60
Aging
  cellulite and, 201–2
  weight gain and, 10, 24–27, **25**
Alcohol, 205
Apathy, weight gain and, 17

Arms, exercises for
  Ab Roller dumbbell curl, 112–13,
    113
  Ab Roller dumbbell overhead press,
    114–15, **115**
  Ab Roller pushups, 108–9, **109**
  dumbbell curl, 96–97
  dumbbell overhead press, 98–99, **99**
  pushups, 92–93, **93**
Asmussen, Erling, 42
Athletic performance, improving, 121
Atrophy of muscles, 27, 165
Average body measurements, 24–25,
  25

B

Back
  exercises for
    Ab Roller dumbbell overhead
      press, 114–15, **115**
    Ab Roller pushups, 108–9, **109**
    dumbbell overhead press, 98–99,
      99
    pushups, 92–93, **93**
  muscles of, 36
Backsliding, 219–20
Barber, Amy, **134**
Beauty, 3–7, 190–92
Before and after photos, 139–40, **140**.
    See also specific participants

tips for, 218
walking, 65–66, 205, 218
External obliques, 36

F

Family. *See* Friends and family
Fat, body
  body weight vs., 13–14
  calories burned by, 22
  cellulite and, 201–2
  function of, 36–37
  hormones and, 32–35
  ideal, 208–9, **208–9**
  measuring, 137–39, 208–9, **208–9**
  muscle-fat cross talk and, 14–16,
    78–79
  muscles turning to, 201
  sleep and, 117, 132
Fat in foods
  daily calories, percentage of, 163
  dieting and, 51–52
  satiety and, 34, 51
  serving sizes of, 164
Fertility, physical indicators of, 4–5
Fiber, 59
15-15-15 negative-accentuated
    training method, 46–47, 132
Fish, 151
Five-part success formula, 18–19
Flat belly exercises, 77–115
  Ab Roller exercises, 100–115
    dumbbell curl, 112–13, **113**
    dumbbell overhead press, 114–15,
      115
    forward crunch, 102–3, **103**
    obliques crunch, 104–5, **105**
    pushups, 108–9, **109**
    squats, 110–11, **111**
    V-crunch, 106–7, **107**
  body weight exercises, 84–95
    forward crunch, 84–87, **85–87**
    obliques crunch, 88–89, **89**
    pushups, 92–93, **93**

    squats, 94–95, **95**
    V-crunch, 90–91, **91**
  dumbbell exercises
    curl, 96–97, **97,** 112–13, **113**
    overhead press, 98–99, **99,**
      114–15, **115**
  guidelines for, 79–82
  inner-ab vacuum, 71–75, **72**
  muscle isolation and, 79
  trouble spots, reducing, 14–16,
    78–79
Flavored floss and toothpaste, <u>216</u>
Flavored water, 214–15
Fluid loss, preventing, 13–14
Foods. *See also* Meals
  carbohydrates in
    daily calories, percentage of, 163
    dieting and, 51–52
    importance of, 54–55, 143,
      193–95
    low-crab diets and, 52, 194–96
    recommendations for, 195
  cravings for
    meal size and, 53
    snacks, 212–13
    taste buds and, <u>216–17</u>
    water consumption to curb,
      205
  eating out, 183–85, 215
  fat in
    daily calories, percentage of, 163
    dieting and, 51–52
    satiety and, 34, 51
    serving sizes of, 164
  preparing for diet, 140–41
  protein in
    calories in, 54
    daily calories, percentage of, 163
    dieting and, 51–52, 194–95
    meal replacement shake, 150
    in meals, 144
    of muscles, 33, 196–98, 201
    vegetarian diets and, 190
  relationship with, 178–80, 183
  texture of, <u>217</u>

Jones, Melissa, **56,** 219
Journal entries
    Jeanenne, water consumption,
        67–69
    Roxanne, personal experience,
        167–87
Journaling, 205, 211, 219

K

Ketone bodies, 194
Kramer, Brianna, **76,** 132, **140,** 190,
    209, 221

L

LaCroix sparkling water, 215
Lassek, Will, 3–4
Legs, exercises for
    Ab Roller squats, 110–11, **111**
    squats, 94–95, **95**
Lennon, Jim, 100
Leptin, 34
Low-calorie treats, 213–14
Low-carbohydrate diets, 52,
    194–96
Lower abdominal muscles, 200
Lunch
    limiting variety of, 144
    week 1–2, <u>145</u>
    week 3–6, 150–51

M

MacCallum, Jennifer, 18, 154, **156,**
    213
Mah, Cheri, 121
Maintenance of weight loss, 34,
    160–66
Manilow, Barry, 157
Maree, Lydia, 100, <u>216–17</u>
Mavrodieva, Elena, **30,** 209

Meals
    composition of, 52
    frequency of, 54
    frozen, 144, 151, 155, 212–13
    inner-ab vacuum exercise before,
        19, 71–75, **72,** 132
    limiting choices for, 144–45,
        155–56
    measuring, 140–41
    sample menu, <u>145–46</u>
    shakes for, 150
    shopping list for, 147
    size of, 19, 32–33, 52–53, 186, 212
    skipping, 53
    walking after, 65
    water before, 59
Measurements, body
    average, 24–25, **25**
    body fat, 137–39, 208–9, **208–9**
    to prepare for diet, 136–39
    updating and evaluating, 165–66
    waist, 14–15, **15,** <u>17</u>
    waist-to-hip ratios, 5, 192–93
    weight, 165
Meat, 147, 151, 164
Media portrayal of women, 3–4, 190
Meditation, 218–19
Meerman, Ruben, 203–4
Melatonin, 219
Menopause, 53
Mental exercises, 81, <u>217</u>
Mentors, 132, 157, 161
Menu, <u>145–46</u>
Metabolism
    age and, 10
    height and, 206
    ketone bodies and, 194
    muscle and, 22
    sleep and, 118–19
Microwave dinners
    dieting and, 52
    menu of, <u>146</u>
    recommendations for, 155, 212–13
    sources of, 144
    300-calorie, 151

T

Tall women, 38, 205–6
Taste buds, <u>216–17</u>
Taylor, Kristi, **40**
Tea, 172
Teeth, <u>216–17</u>
Television before bed, 219
Temperature, body, 38–39, 58, 205, 207
Temptations, 168, 171–72
Test panel. *See also specific participants*
 body fat loss of, 209, **209**
 exercise of, 128, 132, **133**
 journal entries of
  Jeanenne, water consumption, 67–69
  Roxanne, personal experience, 167–87
 organization of, 127–28
 overview, 16, **16,** 18
 six week results of, 130–31
 tips from, 210–21 (*See also* Tips for success)
 twelve week results of, 154
 two vs. six week results, 131–33
 two week results of, 129–30
Texture of food, <u>217</u>
Thighs, body image and, 11
30-30-30 negative-accentuated training method, 45–46
Thulin, Mats, 43–44
Tips for success, 210–21
 adjusting to meals, 212
 backsliding, 219–21
 consistency, <u>220–21</u>
 cravings, 212–13
 desserts, skipping, 213–14
 eating out, 215
 sleeping, 218–19
 sticking to program, 211
 taste buds, training, <u>216–17</u>
 walking, 218
 water consumption, 214–15

Toothpaste, flavored, <u>216</u>
Transverse abdominis, 35–36, 200
Treats, 213–15
Triceps, exercises for
 Ab Roller dumbbell overhead press, 114–15, **115**
 Ab Roller pushups, 108–9, **109**
 dumbbell overhead press, 98–99, **99**
 pushups, 92–93, **93**
Triglycerides, 203
Trombetta, Barbara, **53,** 214–15
Trouble spots, reducing, 78–79
True Lime flavor packets, 214
Tummy, defined, <u>10</u>
Tuna, 151
Twelve week results, 154
Two weeks results, 129–33

U

Urinating
 fat loss through, 59, 203
 increasing from water consumption, 67–69, 170–71

V

Validation, social media and, 11
Variety of meals, 52, 144–45, 155–56
V-crunches, 90–91, **91**
V-crunches, Ab Roller, 106–7, **107**
Vegetables
 adding to frozen dinners, 213
 salads, 151, 215
 serving size of, 164
 shopping list for, 147
 as snacks, 205
Vegetarian diets, 189–90
Virtual Gastric Band Hypnosis, 219
Visualization exercises, 81, <u>217</u>
Vitamins and minerals, 141, 194

W

Waist
average size of, 17
defined, 10
measuring, 14–15, **15**
Waist-to-hip ratio, 4–5, 192–93
Walking for exercise, 65–66, 205, 218
Warming up before exercise, 81
Water consumption
conduction of heat calories and, 38
importance of, 57–61, 60
journal entry example of, 67–69
tips for, 214–15
tracking, 67–68, 214
Water intoxication, 61
Water retention, 58
Waters, Pam, **116,** 212, 215
Water weight, 195
Weather, exercise and, 218
Weeks 1–2, 143–47
limiting choices during, 144–45
menus for, 145–46
power of, 143–44
results after, 129–33
shopping list, 147
workouts for, 80–82, 101
Weeks 3–6
menus for, 149–51
results after, 130–33
workouts for, 81–82, 101
Weight, body
body fat vs., 13–14
components of, 24
measuring, 165, 173

Weight gain
abdominal obesity zone, 17
aging and, 10, 24–27, **25**
of American women, 13
apathy and, 17
dehydration and, 58
Weight loss
capsaicin and, 213
carbohydrates and, 193–96
maintaining, 34
meal size and, 53
recommendations for, 203
science behind, 202–4
sleep and, 117–23 (*See also* Sleep)
of test panel, 128–31, 154, 176, 186
water consumption and, 59, 214–15
water weight, 195
Weights. *See* Dumbbell exercises
Whitney, Eleanor, 50–51

X

X-Force fitness machine, 43–45, **44**

Y

Yang, Yu, **142**